Dermatophytes

THEIR RECOGNITION AND IDENTIFICATION

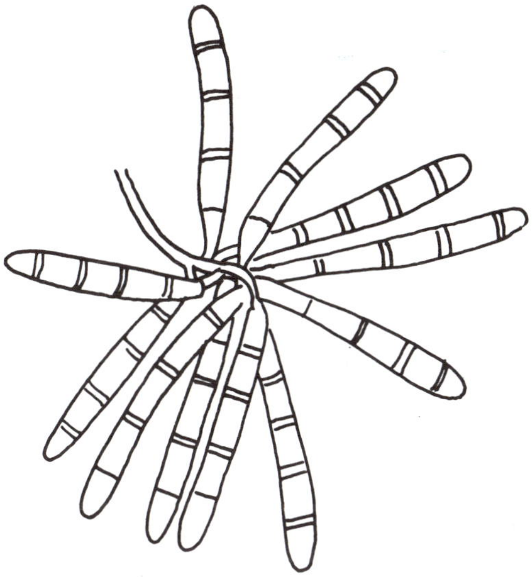

by Gerbert Rebell and David Taplin

UNIVERSITY OF MIAMI PRESS
Coral Gables, Florida

Library of Congress Catalog Card Number
70-130448 ISBN 0-87024-185-0

Studies which have contributed substantially to the information in this manual have been supported in part by the U.S. Army Medical Research and Development Command, Office of the Surgeon General, Washington, D.C. 20315, in cooperation with the Commission on Cutaneous Diseases of the Armed Forces Epidemiological Board.

Production of this manual, including color printing, was subsidized by a generous grant from the Dermatology Foundation of Miami.

Manufactured in the United States of America
by Miami Post

The second edition of this manual

is affectionately dedicated to Harvey Blank,

Professor of Dermatology,

University of Miami School of Medicine

CONTENTS

Contents

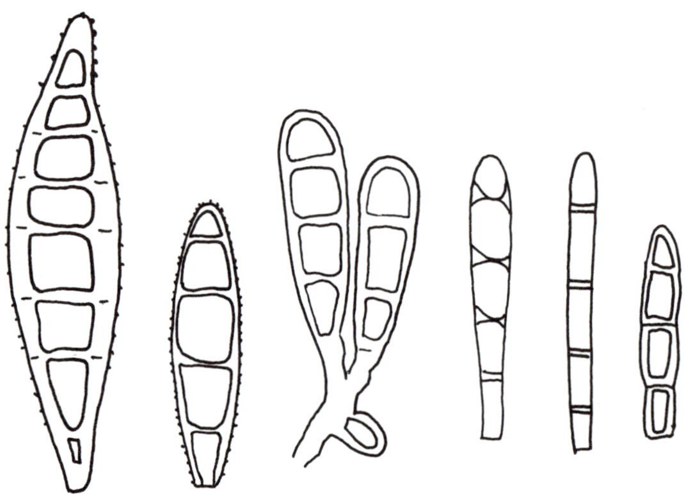

13 23 62 40 50 52

MACROALEURIOSPORES COMMONLY SEEN IN CULTURES FROM HUMAN RINGWORM

PREFACE

This manual attempts to provide an aid in identifying dermatophytes. It was produced in mimeographed form for the American Academy of Dermatology, Chicago, 1963, and in 1964 published in photo-offset with three color plates by the Dermatology Foundation of Miami. The world-wide demand for the manual has exceeded our expectations and actually increased over the years. Reprinting became necessary, so we have taken the opportunity to bring it up to date and make some changes.

Since the first edition the number of recognized species of dermatophytes has increased from twenty-eight to over forty, thirty-two of which have been recorded as producing skin lesions in man. In addition the kinship of the dermatophytes to keratinophilic soil fungi of the genera Arthroderma and Chrysosporium has become apparent. The present edition of the manual has been designed to accommodate these additional species with the least possible disturbance of the grouping and exposition of the 15 or so dermatophytes of paramount importance to human and veterinary medicine.

Because of the larger number of species, the supplementary charts on identification in the first edition have been replaced by a key. The present edition of the manual has a new color plate, showing additional views of common parasitic species and also the new ascigerous species of Microsporum and Trichophyton. Some photographs in the first three plates have been substituted with more representative examples. There is also a page of photomicrographs designed mainly for use with the key.

We have expanded the methods section and have included the new Dermatophyte Test Medium which permits selective isolation and recognition of dermatophytes (and related keratinophylic fungi) without resort to identification of species.

Again, we are indebted to others for consultation and cultures. These include L. Ajello, M.D. Berliner, J.C. Blakemore, H. Böhme, D. Borelli, J.W. Carmichael, M.D. Connole, C.W. Emmons, M.P. English, D. Frey, L.K. Georg, M.A. Gordon, C. Halde, D.W. Mackenzie, M. Marples, G.F. Orr, A.A. Padye, R.S. Pore, J.A. Rioux, J.W. Rippon, S.A. Rosenthal, F.J. Roth, Jr., F.M. Rush-Munro, P.M. Stockdale, R. Vanbreuseghem, and N. Zaias.

We hope once again that we have conveyed something more than a technical interest in these beautiful and fascinating fungi.

Department of Dermatology,
School of Medicine,
University of Miami

GERBERT REBELL
DAVID TAPLIN

August 1st, 1970

Nomenclature

The Emmons-NCDC nomenclature of dermatophytes is used by most workers. Names in recent or present use by the Langeron - Vanbreuseghem school and other sources are included in the index of synonyms at the end of the manual.

In this edition we have replaced the familiar terms macroconidia and microconidia with the larger mouthfuls, macroaleuriospores and microaleuriospores which are mycologically more informative and precise. For similar reasons we have used the terms ascocarp, rather than cleistothecium, and thallus, rather than colony. We hope that the usefulness of the manual will compensate for this outrage.

An aleuriospore is produced by terminal expansion of a hyphal tip, branch, or bud, followed by its disengagement by a septum and somewhat ragged break from the parental hypha.

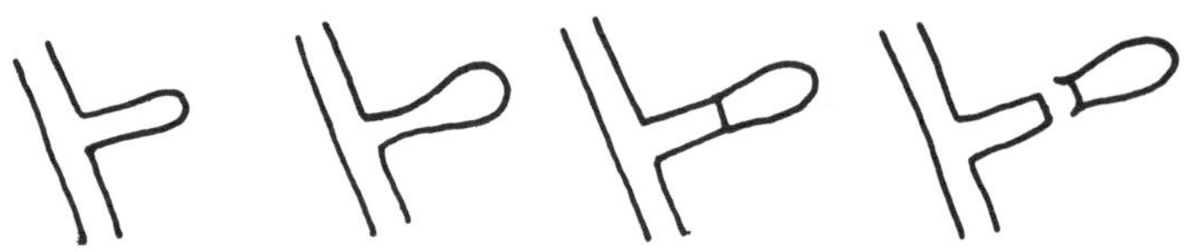

Hints for the Use of the Manual

This manual includes all species of Microsporum, Trichophyton, Epidermophyton, Nannizzia, and Arthroderma, and also fungi with Chrysosporium aleuriospore states which are pertinent to the subject of dermatophytes and their isolation and identification. It is based essentially on a list of authenticated species obtained from publications of the Mycology Unit of the National Communicable Disease Center, U.S. Department of Health and Welfare (Ajello, L., 1968, Sabouraudia 6:147-159).

The manual is designed mainly for the clinical mycologist and veterinarian who needs to identify cultures rapidly, and who normally encounters common pathogens and occasionally a rare or unusual dermatophyte. For human infections we draw attention to: a) the list of known causes of human dermatophytosis on page 10, b) the skeleton outline of the key on page 86 and the designations CHP (common human pathogen) and RHP (rare human pathogen) used throughout the key itself, c) the primary outgrowths of some common dermatophytes illustrated in Plate IV, and d) the drawings of macroaleuriospores on page vi. For veterinary infections we draw attention to: a) the chart listing species encountered in veterinary medicine on page 10 and b) additional notes on pages 22 and 46.

In the introductory pages we have tried to put various aspects of dermatophytes and their identification in a nutshell. The color photographs of typical thalli (pages 75 - 81) should help to identify an unknown culture. Excellent photomicrographs are abundant in the references listed on page 3, and supplement those we have been able to include in the manual on page 83. Throughout the manual black and white drawings are used to delineate salient features.

In the descriptions of species (pages 13 - 71) drawings (particularly in the upper right of each page) depict the most significant common diagnostic features. At the end of each description the critical characteristics are listed on which to base final identification.

It must be expected that strains of dermatophytes will be encountered which cannot be matched with any one of the 54 fungi described here. Most often these are aberrant forms of common species. Until careful comparative taxonomic study made in consultation with an authority such as National Communicable Disease Center (Mycology Unit), Atlanta, Georgia, or Commonwealth Mycological Institute, Ferry Lane, Kew, Surrey, England, an accurate description of the thallus, clinical lesion, and type of hair invasion, etc. is preferable to giving the culture a new name.

Standard References

Where illustrative material is not available in one or more of these standard references, additional references will be given following descriptions of each species.

AJELLO, l., GEORG, L.K., KAPLAN, W., and KAUFMAN, L.: Laboratory Manual for Medical Mycology, Public Health Service Publication No. 994. U.S. Government Printing Office, Washington, D.C. (1963). (Revised edition in preparation).

CONANT, N.H., SMITH, D.T., BAKER, R.D., and CALLOWAY, J.L.: Manual of Clinical Mycology, W.B. Saunders Co., Philadelphia, Pa. 3rd Edition (1962).

EMMONS, C.W., BINFORD, C.H., and UTZ, J.P.: Medical Mycology, Lea & Febiger, Philadelphia, Pa. (1963). (Revised edition in preparation).

GÖTZ, H.: Die Pilzkrankheiten der Haut durch Dermatophyten (Handbuch der Haut-und Geschlechtskrankheiten, J. Jaddassohn, Ergänzungswerk, IV/3), Springer-Verlag, Berlin-Göttingen-Heidelberg, Germany (1962).

HAZEN, E.L., GORDON, M.A., and REED, F.C.: Laboratory Identification of Pathogenic Fungi Simplified. Charles C. Thomas, Springfield, Ill. 3rd Edition (1970).

LEWIS, G.M., HOPPER, M.E., WILSON, J.W., and PLUNKETT, O.A.: An Introduction to Medical Mycology. The Year Book Publishers, Inc., Chicago, Ill., 4th Edition (1958).

DVORAK, J. and OTCENASEK, M.: Mycological Diagnosis of Animal Dermatophytosis. Academia, Prague (1969).

The Review of Medical and Veterinary Mycology, an annotated bibliography published quarterly by the Commonwealth Mycological Institute, Kew, England, has been of great value in the preparation of this manual, and is recommended as a source of current information, listed mainly under "Dermatomycetes".

We regret that limitations of space and cost have not permitted us to include specific references to the many publications on the dermatophytes which have been used without acknowledgement in preparing the text of this manual. The references we have cited are limited specifically to those which aid in recognizing and identifying dermatophyte species.

Epidemiology and Ecology

The dermatophytes may be thought of as a group of taxonomically related fungi with affinity for cornified epidermis, hair, horn, nails, and feathers. Many, perhaps all, digest keratin substrates enzymatically. When present in soil, they are among those fungi which are referred to as keratinophilic because they can be isolated from hair, feathers, etc., placed as "bait" in contact with the soil. The species of dermatophytes may be categorized as geophilic, zoophilic, and anthropophilic.

Geophilic dermatophytes are those which inhabit soil where they probably decompose keratinous debris. In this manual we class a minimum of five species of Microsporum and six species of Trichophyton as geophilic. Chrysosporium species are also predominantly geophilic and those which appear to be related to dermatophytes are keratinophilic. Geophilic species are also frequently isolated from the hair of small wild mammals in the absence of lesions. Other natural sources include birds, bird nests, and the soil around animal burrows. T. terrestre and Chrysosporium indicum and tropicum are frequently isolated as contaminants on the human skin and might be confused with T. mentagrophytes.

Zoophilic dermatophytes are those primarily parasitic on animals other than man. We have classed nine species as zoophilic. Of these: M. nanum may proliferate in soil and therefore be equally well classed as geophilic, but is not isolated from soil except in pig yards. T. simii also occurs in soil and dropped feathers, and perhaps should be classified as geophilic, but its geographical restriction to India suggests that it may depend on an endemic animal. T. mentagrophytes and T. erinacei do not thrive in soil, possibly because of bacterial attack, and M. persicolor although locally abundant in Europe on the fur of small mammals has never been isolated from soil. Lesions with T. erinacei in the hedgehog, T. mentagrophytes in Rattus, and M. persicolor in the Bank Vole may be associated with epidermal mites suggesting the possibility of a symbiotic or dependent relationship between the fungi and the mites. All of the known zoophilic dermatophytic fungi sometimes produce infections in man.

Anthropophilic dermatophytes are those which are primarily parasitic on man. Man is host to twelve strictly parasitic anthropophilic species, most of which exhibit reduced sporulation in culture and apparently depend on arthrospores produced in scalp hairs and desquamating human epidermis for dissemination. In particular, two groups of parasitic species, the small-spored Microsporums and the endothrix Trichophytons appear to have evolved specialized types of sporulation in infected hair which allow dissemination and contagion. One species, Trichophyton concentricum may be suspected of having evolved a similar mechanism through a specialized type of induced epidermal scaling.

Geographical Distribution and Variation

Geophilic dermatophytes apparently occur world-wide in appropriate soils. Zoophilic and anthropophilic species exhibit three types of geographical localization: (1) Some zoophilic species appear to be geographically restricted to the range of a preferred animal host as, for example, M. persicolor and T. erinacei, (2) Among anthropophilic species there are marked geographical patterns, such as in the distribution of species which cause ectothrix and endothrix scalp infections, and in the virtually anthropological association of T. concentricum with primitive cultures of the Pacific Islands, South Asia, and neotropics, (3) Widely distributed species may have regional variants. For example, isolates of T. equinum in Australia and New Zealand do not have the requirement for nicotinic acid which characterizes the species elsewhere.

The restricted geographical occurrence of T. megnini and T. simii, two fairly well known species, is presently inexplicable.

Hair Invasion in Culture and in Soil

Many geophilic and zoophilic dermatophytes characteristically perforate hair in vitro by means of special hyphal appendages called perforating organs. Other species erode the hair cuticle but may not form perforating structures. Under controlled conditions (see methods) perforation of hair appears to be a reliable way of differentiating T. mentagrophytes from T. rubrum.

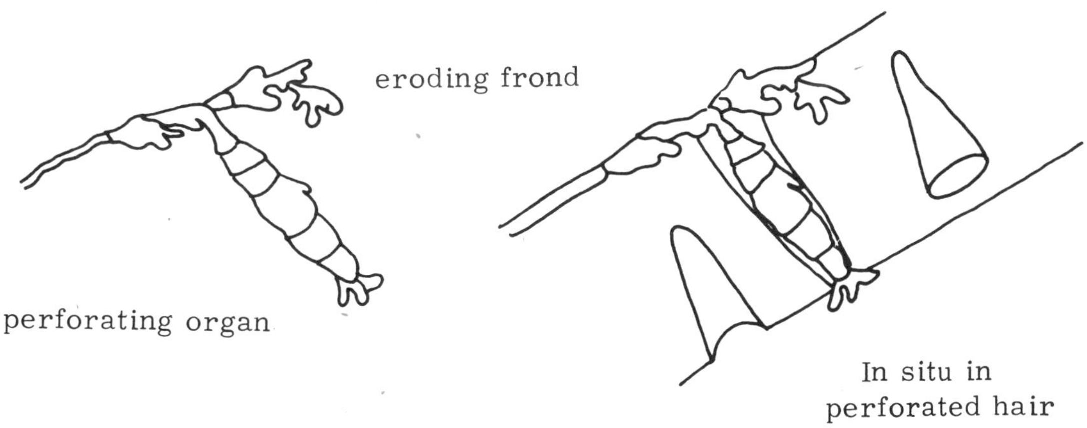

Properties Useful in Isolation and Recognition

Dermatophytes, in addition to having distinctive macro- and microaleuriospores, causing ringworm lesions, and having a predilection for keratinous substrates, are along with keratinophilic species of Chrysosporium and other apparently related fungi, also characterized by: (1) production of and tolerance of an alkaline pH in culture media, (2) sensitivity to 20 $\mu g/ml$ or less of griseofulvin, and (3) resistance to 500 $\mu g/ml$ of cycloheximide. This combination of properties sets them apart from many other fungi and permits the design of culture media and techniques for their selective isolation and recognition.

Infections in Man

In addition to the anthropophilic species, all zoophilic and at least six geophilic species of dermatophytes have been reported to cause tinea corporis in man (usually also tinea capitis). The six are N. incurvata, N. gypsea, M. fulvum, M. vanbreuseghemii, M. cookei, and T. vanbreuseghemii. To this we could add the presumptive geophilic species M. praecox, T. proliferans, and also M. nanum and T. simii which we arbitrarily have classed as zoophilic in this manual. In general lesions produced in man by geophilic and zoophilic species are more eczematous or inflammatory and less chronic than those produced by anthropophilic species. In rare patients dermatophyte infections may be overwelming and granulomatous or invasive. This has been reported with T. rubrum, M. canis, E. floccosum, T. tonsurans, T. schoenleinii, and other species. A table of clinical types of dermatophytosis is given on page 10.

Hair Parasitism

In tinea capitis and tinea barbae and less obviously in tinea corporis, there is parasitism of the living hair. In this process the vegetative growth of hyphae occurs within the hair above the zone of keratinization of the hair shaft and keeps pace with the growth of hair. Distal to this zone of active growth, arthrospores are formed within or on the surface of the hair by most species of dermatophytes. The location and size of the arthrospores constitute important differences in the classification of dermatophytes. Among parasitic species, E. floccosum, T. concentricum, and M. persicolor are not known to parasitize hair. A table of types of hair parasitism is given on page 12.

Hair Fluorescence

In tinea capitis caused by the parasitic Microsporum species (M. canis, M. distortum, M. audouinii, and M. ferrugineum) the parasitized hairs are usually but not always brightly fluorescent yellow-green. Human hairs parasitized by other dermatophytes are very rarely if ever fluorescent, except for T. schoenleinii where dull bluish-white fluorescence is frequent. However, fluorescence is dependent on the host animal as well as on the dermatophyte species. The fluorescence of hair with dermatophyte infections appears to be due to tryptophan metabolites.

Genetic Instability (Pleomorphism)

Most dermatophyte thalli regularly undergo fluffy degenerative changes in laboratory culture with loss of identifying aleuriospores and pigments. Subcultures of thalli especially those on Sabouraud Dextrose Agar must be made frequently and selectively to maintain the characteristic features. These changes have been shown to be due to mutation and chromosome aberrations. M. audouinii and T. megninii appear to be genetically more stable in culture than other dermatophytes.

Special Nutritional Requirements

A number of the parasitic dermatophytes have essential or partial nutritional requirements which help to identify them. Important examples are T. verrucosum (thiamine and inositol), T. megninii (l-histidine), T. equinum (niacin), and T. tonsurans and T. violaceum (thiamine), see: Georg, L. K., 1957. Routine Nutritional Tests for the Identification of Dermatophytes, J. Bact. 74:113-121.

Appearance of Thallus (Colony)

The thalli of dermatophytes are either (a) flat and more or less fluffy, or (b) slow-growing, heaped and folded and more or less glabrous. Many may have cream to buff powdery surfaces due to the presence of macro- and/ or microaleuriospores. Many thalli develop non-diffusing red or yellow pigments. These pigments are mostly chromatic variations of the same chemical substances, often with a greenish melanoid hue. A few species or isolates produce red, yellow, dark brown, or blue-black pigments which diffuse into the medium.

Media enriched with vitamins, e.g. yeast extract, produce folded and more compact thalli in the case of most dermatophytes. The appearance of typical thalli of the important species is shown in the color photographs, page 75.

Microscopic Morphology

Most dermatophytes have two types of aleuriospores: multicelled macroaleuriospores and small microaleuriospores. Macroaleuriospores of the genus Microsporum tend to have rough walls; those of Trichophyton and Epidermophyton have smooth walls. Macroaleuriospores of M. vanbreuseghemii, T. (M?) gallinae, M. persicolor, and M. audouinii often appear to be smooth walled. In these species growth in soil and hair seems to promote rough walled macroaleuriospores.

Microaleuriospores are produced by most dermatophytes on occasion. Among pathogenic species Epidermophyton floccosum is unique in that although macroaleuriospores are abundant, microaleuriospores are never produced. Microaleuriospores of the parasitic Microsporum species are often relatively slender and stick-like. Microaleuriospores are used in the identification of several species; notably M. persicolor, T. mentagrophytes, T. tonsurans, T. rubrum, T. terrestre, T. georgiae, T. phaseoliforme, and various species of Chrysosporium (photomicrographs, page 83).

Other microscopic structures have little or no diagnostic value. Exceptions are: (1) terminal chlamydospores and pectinate hyphae in M. audouinii, (2) "nail head" antler hyphae in T. schoenleinii, (3) spirals in the presence of abundant spherical microaleuriospores in T. mentagrophytes, (4) arthrospores and reflexive branching in T. soudanense, (5) nodular organs in T. mentagrophytes var nodulare, (6) "propagules" in T. proliferans, and (7) pycnidia-like structures in T. phaseoliforme.

The Perfect Ascigerous State

"A pinch of dirt, a wisp of hair,
And thou beside me in the petri dish!"

Most of the soil inhabiting dermatophytes and to date four of the zoophilic species develop ascocarps (cleistothecia) containing ascospores which place them in the ascomycetes. These are obtained by mating two compatible isolates on a substrate of soil and hair. There are two perfect genera: Nannizzia (for Microsporum) and Arthroderma (for Trichophyton and some species of Chrysosporium) which are distinguished by the morphology of the peridial hyphae forming the ascocarp structure (see below). Two geophilic species, A. curreyi and A. georgiae and possibly some isolates of T. mentagrophytes are homothallic (produce fertile ascocarps without mating). Structures suggestive of ascocarps and peridial hyphae, often associated with microaleuriospores but without ascospores, are seen in unmated cultures of heterothallic dermatophytes and also in T. rubrum and other species where the perfect state has not yet been found. These probably indicate an inherent capacity to mate under suitable conditions or vestigial evidence of the same.

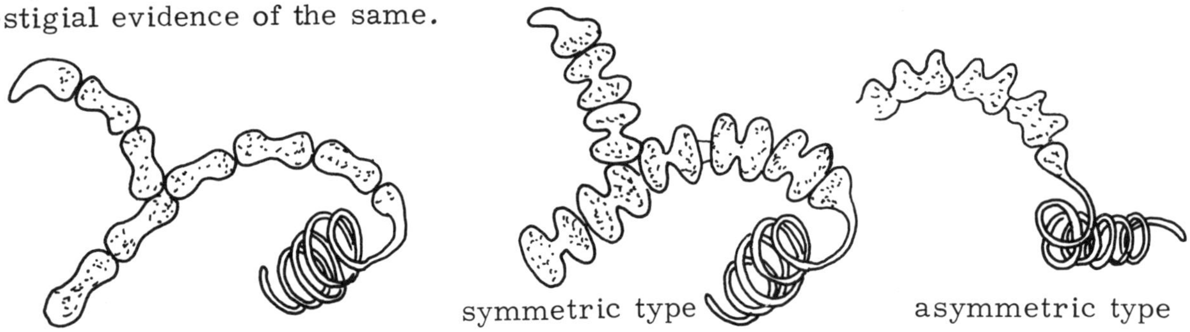

symmetric type asymmetric type

Nannizzia Arthroderma

The intricacies of this interesting subject are beyond the scope of this manual. However, the relationship of the perfect state of ascigerous dermatophytes to the conidial types may be illustrated as follows:

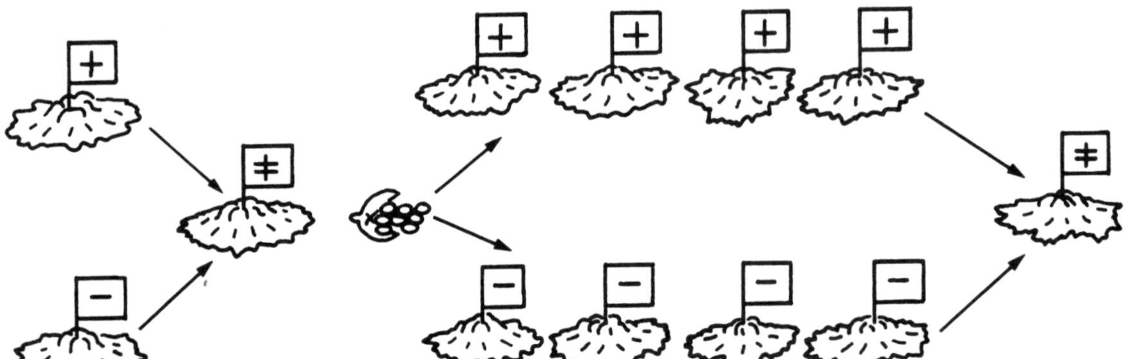

(A) (B) (C) (D)

Two thalli of Microsporum gypseum (A) of opposite "sex" come into proximity with each other and join to form thallus of Nannizzia incurvata (B) which produced asci, each containing eight ascospores. The eight ascospores germinate, producing eight new strains of Microsporum gypseum (C), new because of the genetic recombinations occurring in the production of the ascospores. These eight strains of Microsporum gypseum consist of four strains of each "sex". Strains of opposite "sex" if they chance to meet unite to form a new thallus of Nannizzia incurvata (D). The terms male and female are not usually applied to fungi. The terms "+" and "-" are used instead, to indicate strains which copulate and which are said to be opposite or compatible mating types. They may also be designated by "A" and "a", signifying that mating type is determined by genetic alleles.

A similar diagram can be drawn for other ascigerous dermatophytes. Strains of Microsporum gypseum derived from Nannizzia gypsea will not mate with strains derived from Nannizzia incurvata. There are, thus, two species of Ascomycetes which manifest the conidial form of Microsporum gypseum. This is a common situation in mycology. The existence of two systems of nomenclature, one applying to the perfect state, and the other to the conidial state is required because many molds are known only by their conidial forms.

The international rules governing nomenclature of fungi stipulate that the name associated with the perfect state should be used and should supercede the name of the conidial state. For example, M. gypseum should be referred to as Nannizzia incurvata; or as N. incurvata, Microsporum state; or as N. incurvata (+); etc.; all which are acceptable combinations. However, in this manual we use perfect state designations only for laboratory cultures which have been test mated, since it is difficult or impossible to identify some perfect species in their conidial forms (see M. gypseum and T. terrestre).

Mating Types

The mating types of both ascigerous and imperfect dermatophytes may frequently be identified by their reaction to physical contact with the mating types of Arthroderma simii (see methods, page 117). Using this method of determination, it appears that strictly parasitic species, such as T. rubrum, M. audouinii, and T. erinacei may be represented in nature by only one mating type. It has been observed that in ascigerous dermatophytes, such as T. mentagrophytes, one mating type may be associated with more inflammatory lesions than the other. Exclusion of one mating type by natural selection in the evolution of strictly parasitic species is therefore a tenable hypothesis, since well-adapted parasitism is classically associated with tolerance of the parasite by the host. In ascigerous dermatophytes which display differences between the pathogenic properties of the two mating types, enzyme activities, such as elastase and urease, appear to be genetically linked to the mating type associated with inflammatory lesions. Such findings also make it advisable to determine the mating types of dermatophytes used in experimental studies.

"When A doth meet his ideal mate
a ends up in the perfect state !"

MAJOR EPIDEMIOLOGICAL CLASSES OF HUMAN DERMATOPHYTE INFECTIONS

Epidemic usually fluorescent tinea capitis and associated tinea corporis

16 M. audouinii (anthropophilic - commonest in Africa, Europe, and America)
19 M. ferrugineum (anthropophilic - commonest in Africa, Balkans, and Asia)

Sporadic usually fluorescent tinea capitis and associated tinea corporis

13 M. canis (zoophilic - widespread and common)
15 M. distortum (zoophilic - local and rare)

Epidemic non-fluorescent tinea capitis and associated tinea corporis

52 T. tonsurans (anthropophilic - commonest in Europe and America)
54 T. violaceum (anthropophilic - commonest in Africa and Eurasia)
55 T. gourvilii (anthropophilic - Africa)
56 T. soudanense (anthropophilic - Africa)
58 T. yaoundei (anthropophilic - Africa)

Epidemic favus - scutula and scaling forms

59 T. schoenleinii (anthropophilic - commonest in Eurasia and North Africa)

Epidemic tinea corporis

62 E. floccosum (anthropophilic - world-wide)
50 T. rubrum (anthropophilic - world-wide)
61 T. concentricum (anthropophilic - South Pacific and Tropical America)
40 T. mentagrophytes (zoophilic - Vietnam, Southeast Asia)

Epidemic tinea pedis and intertriginous tinea corporis

50 T. rubrum (anthropophilic - world-wide)
40 T. mentagrophytes (anthropophilic form- world-wide) mainly tinea pedis
62 E. floccosum (anthropophilic - world-wide)

Epidemic tinea barbae and associated tinea corporis and tinea capitis

49 T. megninii (anthropophilic - Europe)

Rare tinea capitis and tinea barbae, common as tinea corporis

50 T. rubrum (anthropophilic - world-wide)

Frequent but sporadic tinea corporis, tinea capitis, and tinea barbae

40 T. mentagrophytes (zoophilic and possibly geophilic - world-wide)
47 T. verrucosum (zoophilic - world-wide)
23 M. gypseum (geophilic -world-wide)
38 T. simii (zoophilic - India) only tinea corporis
44 T. erinacei (zoophilic - New Zealand) also endemic in Europe

Rare, sporadic tinea corporis, tinea capitis, and tinea barbae

25 M. fulvum (geophilic - world-wide)
27 M. persicolor (zoophilic - Europe and Africa) only tinea corporis
26 M. nanum (zoophilic - world-wide)
64 M. praecox (geophilic? - Europe?)
21 T. (M?) gallinae (zoophilic - world-wide)
30 M. vanbreuseghemii (geophilic - world-wide)
29 M. cookei (geophilic - world-wide)
45 T. equinum (zoophilic -world-wide)
67 T. proliferans (? -- Great Britain, New Zealand)
37 T. vanbreuseghemii (geophilic - world-wide)
69 T. fluviomuniense (? -- Africa?)
31 T. ajelloi (geophilic - world-wide) questionable pathogenicity

DERMATOPHYTES IN VETERINARY PRACTICE

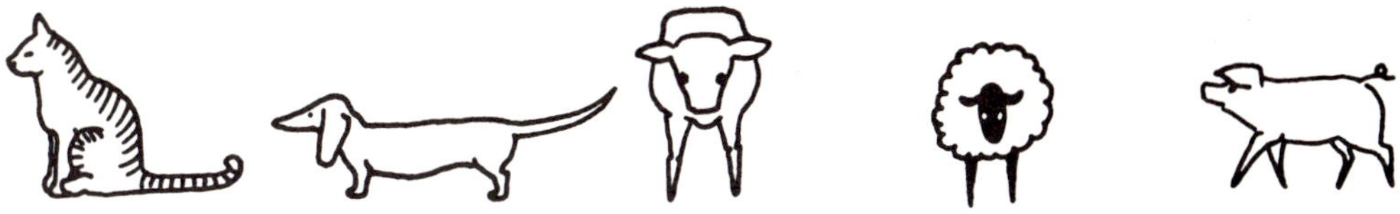

13	M. canis	usual	frequent	reported	occasional	reported
15	M. distortum	reported	reported	-	-	-
16	M. audouinii	-	reported	-	-	-
21	T. (M?) gallinae	reported	reported	-	-	-
23	M. gypseum	occasional	frequent	reported	-	reported
26	M. nanum	-	-	-	-	usual
27	M. persicolor	-	reported	-	-	-
29	M. cookei	-	reported	-	-	-
30	M. vanbreuseghemii	-	reported	-	-	-
31	T. ajelloi	-	questionable	questionable	-	-
38	T. simii	-	reported	-	-	-
40	T. mentagrophytes	occasional	frequent	occasional	occasional	occasional
45	T. equinum	-	reported	-	-	-
47	T. verrucosum	reported	reported	usual	occasional	reported
49	T. megninii	-	reported	-	-	-
50	T. rubrum	-	reported	-	-	-
54	T. violaceum	reported	-	-	-	-
62	E. floccosum	-	reported	-	-	-

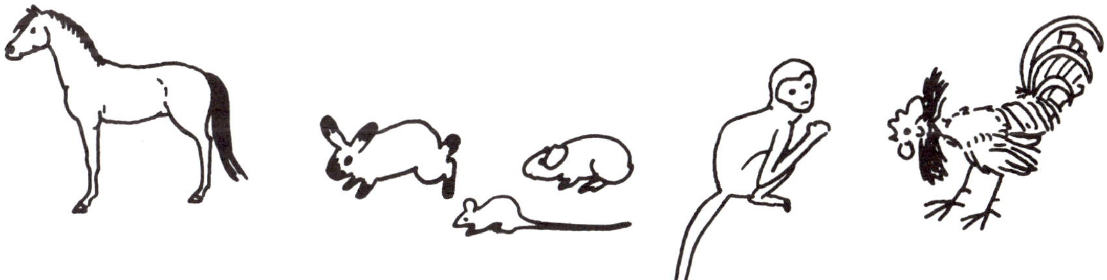

13	M. canis	occasional	occasional	frequent	-
15	M. distortum	reported	-	reported	-
16	M. audouinii	-	-	reported	-
21	T. (M?) gallinae	-	reported	reported	usual
23	M. gypseum	frequent	frequent	occasional	-
29	M. cookei	-	-	reported	-
30	M. vanbreuseghemii	-	reported	-	-
31	T. ajelloi	questionable	-	-	-
38	T. simii	-	-	frequent (India)	frequent (India)
40	T. mentagrophytes	occasional	usual	frequent	-
45	T. equinum	usual	-	-	-
47	T. verrucosum	occasional	-	-	-
50	T. rubrum	-	-	reported	-

There are reports of T. schoenleinii infections in animals and birds where this fungus is common.

PARASITIZED HUMAN HAIR

I. Ectothrix (Spores outside hair shaft (2-3 microns)

Small spores (microsporum) (not clearly visible with low power objective) in masses. Hair usually brightly fluorescent, Fig. 1.

13 M. canis
16 M. audouinii
15 M. distortum
19 M. ferrugineum

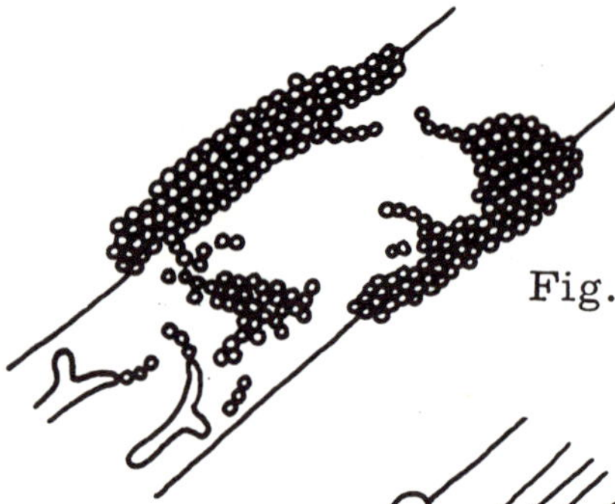

Fig. 1

Large spores, 5-8 microns in sparse chains inside and outside of hair (visible with lower power objective). Hair not fluorescent, Fig. 2.

23 M. gypseum
25 M. fulvum
26 M. nanum
30 M. vanbreuseghemii
21 T. (M?) gallinae

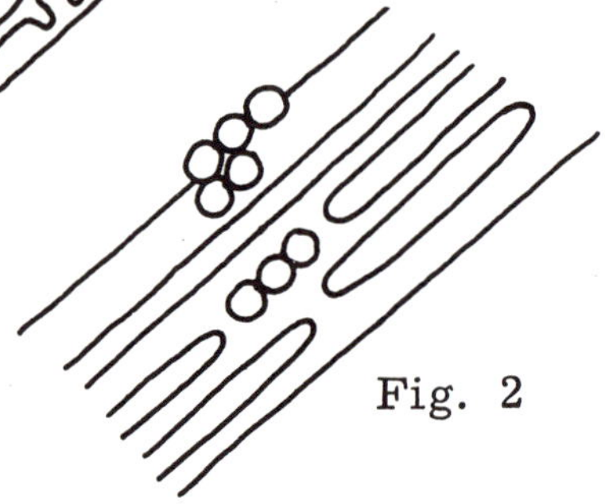

Fig. 2

Large spores in chains (Trichophyton) (visible with low power objective). Hair not fluorescent.

megaspore type (5-10 microns), Fig. 3.
47 T. verrucosum

microides type (3-5 microns), Fig. 4.
40 T. mentagrophytes

intermediate types
50 T. rubrum (reported)
49 T. megninii

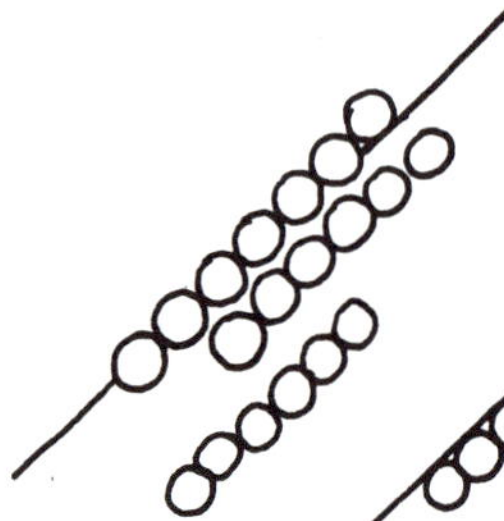

Fig. 3

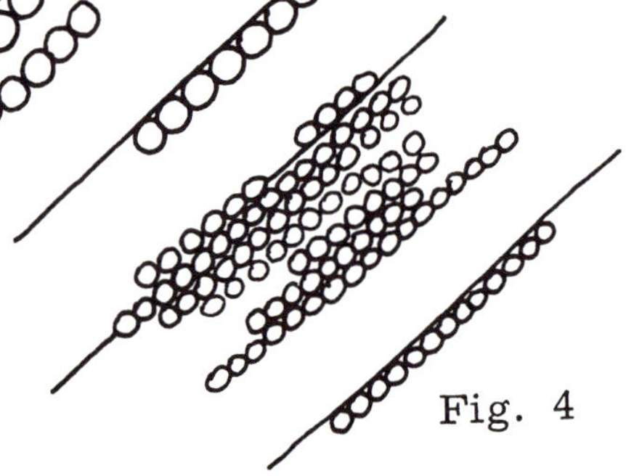

Fig. 4

II. Endothrix - (Spores (5-8 microns) inside hair shaft - hairs break off short and curl), Fig. 5.

52 T. tonsurans
54 T. violaceum
56 T. soudanense
58 T. yaoundei
55 T. gourvilii
50 T. rubrum (reported)

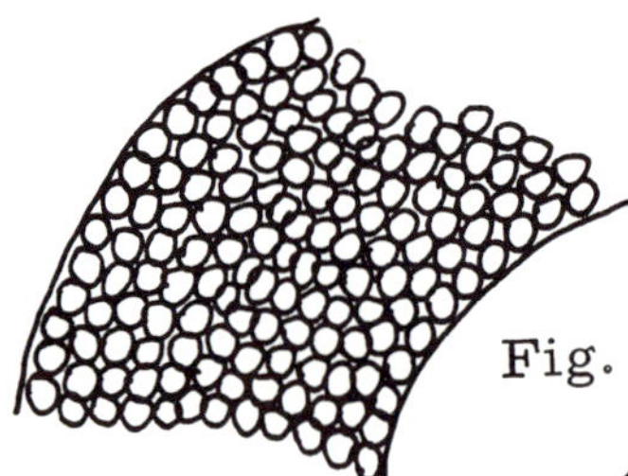

Fig. 5

III. Hyphae and air spaces but usually no spores in hair, dull fluorescence - hairs remain long, Fig. 6.

59 T. schoenleinii

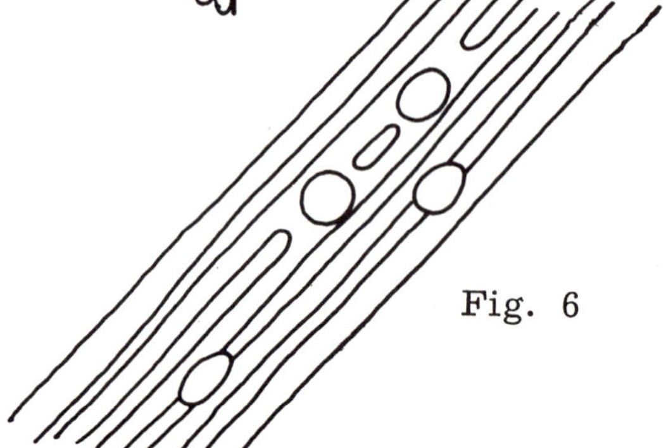

Fig. 6

IV. No parasitism of hair.

61 T. concentricum
62 Epidermophyton floccosum
27 M. persicolor

Identification of Microsporum canis

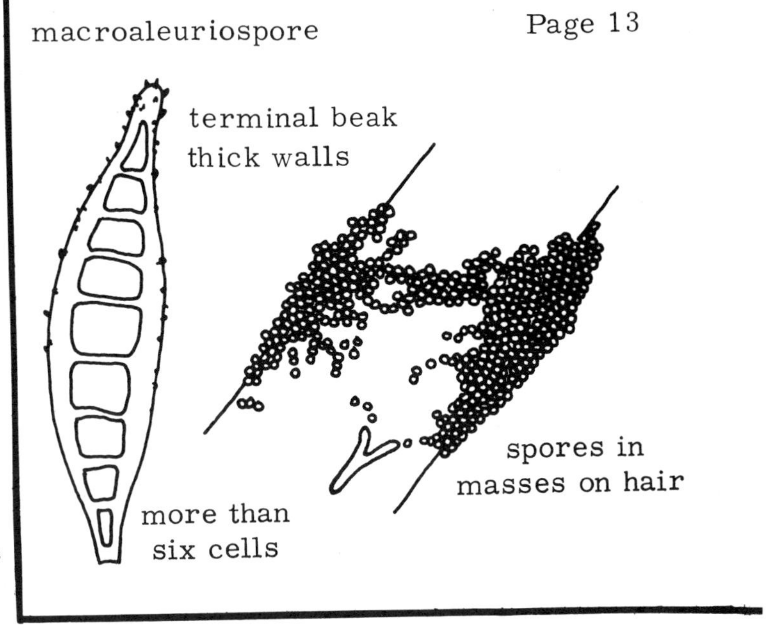

Invasion of Hair - Sporulation ectothrix in masses produced from profuse branching hyphae which ensheath the hair shaft. Spores are small and require the high dry (40X) objective to be discerned. Hairs usually, but not always, brightly fluoresce due to a metabolite produced by the fungus in the hair.

Clinical Disease - Typically tinea capitis and tinea corporis, most prevalent in children. Generalized infections and onychomycosis have been reported. Usually more inflammatory and less chronic than M. audouinii with a greater incidence of tinea corporis. In cat, crusting or non-inflammatory lesions particularly on nose and feet become chronic and subclinical, but revealed by presence of fluorescent hairs.

Epidemiology - The cat ringworm. Infections can usually be traced to a neighborhood pet. Dogs are frequently infected also. See page 22.

Geographical Distribution - World-wide. Perhaps the most generally distributed type of tinea capitis. Uncommon in equatorial Africa.

Appearance of Thallus - A whitish, coarsely fluffy, spreading thallus which usually develops a characteristic deep yellow pigment on the underside. In texture M. canis is distinctly more hairy than M. audouinii. Radial grooves are more closely spaced. Cottony tufts develop as the thallus matures. Diffuse fluffy pleomorphism occurs rather early. The yellow color develops in the first week of thallus growth and becomes dull and hard to discern in old thalli. On potato dextrose agar the pigment is lemon yellow, but easily seen because of the sparse development of aerial hyphae. Primary isolates (called dysgonic) may be glabrous, heaped, and deeply pigmented with distorted, pigmented hyphae, suggestive of M. ferrugineum, but typically fluffy sections with macroaleuriospores usually quickly develop in culture. Plates I and IV.

Microscopic Morphology - Macroaleuriospores are usually produced in fair numbers and are characteristic. They are long, spindle-shaped, frequently thick-walled, usually with an asymmetrical knob. The rough surface of the macroaleuriospore is particularly evident at the knob. Usually more than six compartments. The slenderness of the macroaleuriospores and the length of the terminal knob vary considerably from strain to strain. Slender clavate to pyriform microaleuriospores may be seen but are not diagnostic of the species.

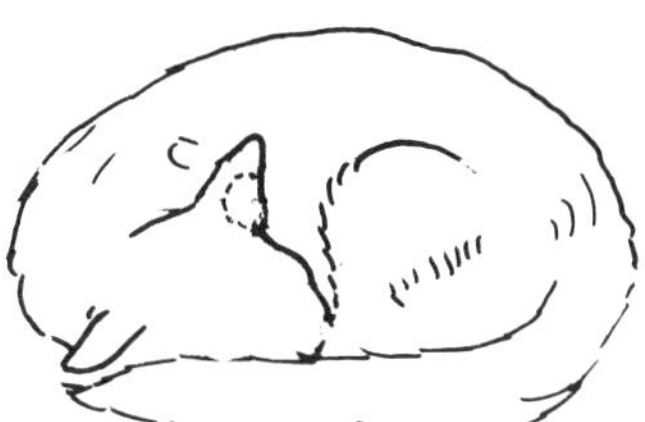

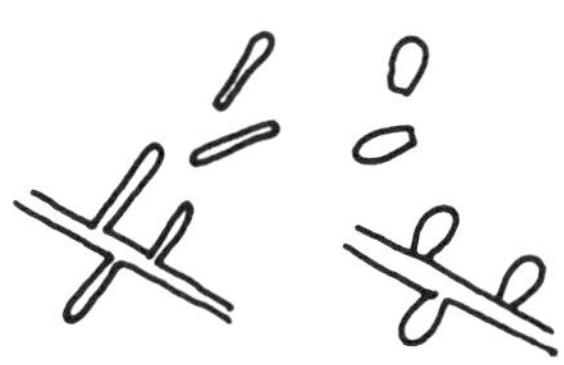

microaleuriospores

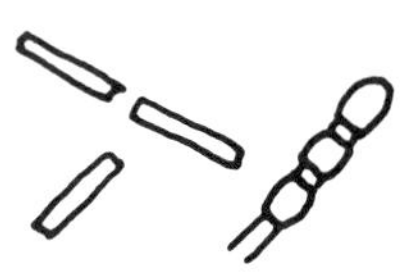

arthroaleuriospores

Microsporum canis - Cont.

Special Nutritional Requirements - None reported. Unlike M. audouinii, M. canis grows profusely on polished rice.

Variants - Strains of M. canis which fail to produce yellow pigment are occasionally encountered. So called dysgonic strains are obtained which are initially slow-growing and may cease to grow entirely, or may have poorly developed macro-aleuriospores (var. obesum). Microscopic morphology and growth on polished rice are the features most to be relied upon. Possibly there are varieties of M. canis which are native to monkeys and apes (especially var. obesum) and in certain regions to horses (var. equinum), as distinct from infections in these animals with the common feline form. A variant producing abundant micro-aleuriospores has been isolated from beach soil in Romania.

Perfect State - Unknown.

Special Media - In distinguishing M. canis from M. audouinii both polished rice media and potato agar are helpful. On potato dextrose agar, M. audouinii usually produces a salmon and M. canis a yellow pigment beneath the thallus.

Critical Characteristics - (1) Characteristic macroaleuriospores, (2) Yellow pigment.

References:

Johnstone, K.I. and LaTouche, C.J., 1956. Cultural Characteristics of Dysgonic Strains of Microsporum canis Bodin, Trans. Brit. Mycol. Soc. 39:442-448.

Klokke, A.H. and deVries, G.A., 1963. Tinea capitis in Chimpanzees Caused by Microsporum canis Bodin 1902 Resembling M. obesum Conant 1937, Sabouraudia 2:268-270.

Evolceanu, R. and Alteraş, I., 1967. Isolierung von Microsporum canis aus Bodenproben in Rumanien (Bukarest), Mykosen 10:243-246.

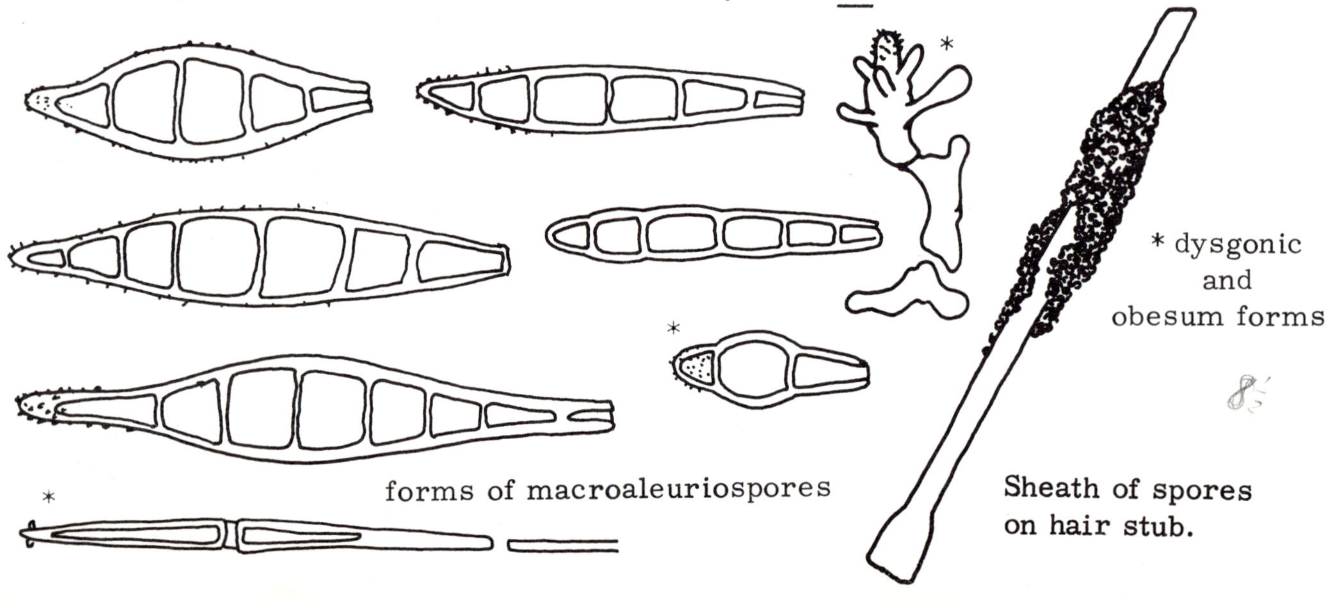

Identification of Microsporum distortum

Invasion of Hair - Identical to M. canis. Usually fluorescent.

Clinical Disease - Similar to M. canis.

Epidemiology - An uncommon cause of Microsporum tinea capitis, so far reported principally from South Island of New Zealand and from Australia in rural areas. Cases have been described from the United States and traced to contact with pet South American monkeys. Infections in cats, dogs, and other animals occur. The natural reservoir of the species is unknown. Possibly a variant of M. canis.

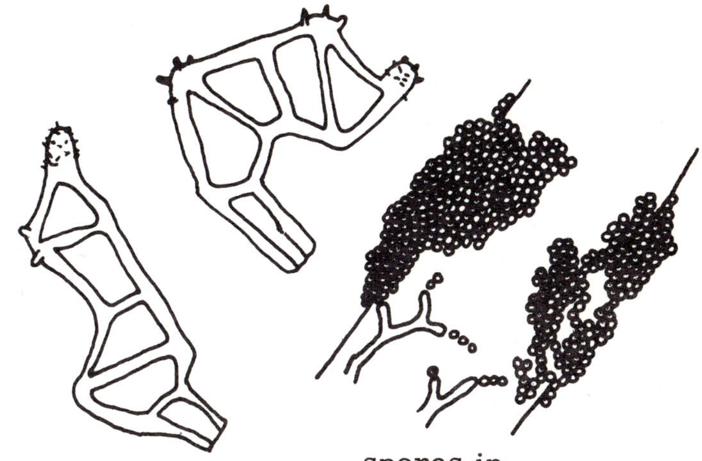

Geographical Distribution - So far reported from Australia, New Zealand and the United States. Potentially world wide.

Appearance of Thallus - New Zealand isolates usually resemble M. canis but with little pigment production *. A strain isolated in the United States is slow growing, flat, densely fuzzy, with a moderate amount of yellow on the undersurface of the thallus and large numbers of microaleuriospores **. A sparse buff powdery surface may be present if aleuriospores are numerous. Plate I.

Microscopic Morphology - Macroaleuriospores resembling those of M. canis but grossly bent and distorted in shape. Clavate microaleuriospores often abundant (an uncommon finding in M. canis).

Special Nutritional Requirements - None reported.

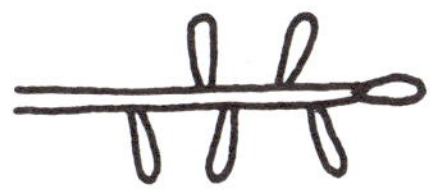

Variants - Thallus may be spreading with little pigment production or compact and yellowish white.

Perfect State - Not known.

Special Media - Like M. canis growth and sporulation abundant on polished rice.

Critical Characteristics - (1) Macroaleuriospores.

References:

* Marples, M.J. and Smith, J.M.B., 1962. Further Observations on the Ecology of Microsporum distortum, New Zealand Medical Journal, 61:539-544.

Frey, D. and Flood, J., 1968. Ringworm in a Child Due to Microsporum distortum, Aust. J. Dermat. 9:218-220.

** Kaplan, W., Georg, L.K., Hendricks,S.L.and Leeper, R.A., 1957. Isolation of Microsporum distortum from Animals in the United States, J. Invest. Dermat., 28:449-453.

Identification of Microsporum audouinii

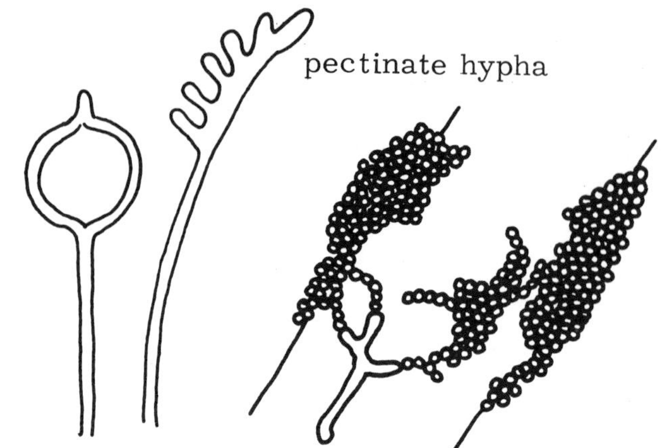

Invasion of Hair - Invasion of hair is identical to that seen in M. canis. Infected hairs are usually, but not always brightly fluorescent.

Clinical Disease - Typical tinea capitis and tinea corporis, most prevalent in children. Usually less inflammatory and more chronic than M. canis. Kerion may occur. Lesions on the glabrous skin are less frequent than with M. canis.

Epidemiology - Epidemic tinea capitis of prepubertal years. Notable outbreaks in major cities of North America and Europe. Increasing in rural areas, probably as a result of regional schools. Essentially restricted to man, although infections have been reported in the dog and monkeys. In some cases these have been caused by atypical strains of doubtful classification. See page 22.

Geographical Distribution - World-wide in urban and quasi-urban areas.

Appearance of Thallus - Characteristically flat spreading and dense, with greyish or slightly tannish white surfaces, suggesting mouse fur in texture. Some salmon or peach color pigment is formed under the central portion of the thallus. This is best seen on potato dextrose agar. In contrast to T. mentagrophytes the thallus of M. audouinii is less dense and more appressed and spreading. Plates I and IV

Microscopic Morphology - Colonies of M. audouinii are usually almost devoid of spore forms. Characteristic terminal chlamydospores are usually present and are a fairly safe diagnostic feature. Occasional strains produce macroaleuriospores which may resemble those of M. canis but usually are longer, smoother and poorly shaped. Microaleuriospores, usually absent, are identical to those seen in other Microsporum species. Pectinate hyphae cited in older literature are seen in some isolates of M. audouinii on routine media and characterize var. rivalieri. Terminal chlamydospores are seen also in T. tonsurans and pectinate hyphae in T. rubrum, but these species usually have abundant and characteristic microaleuriospores.

Special Nutritional Requirements - Nutritional studies of M. audouinii have failed to reveal requirements common to all strains. Unlike M. canis, however, M. audouinii grows very poorly on polished rice.

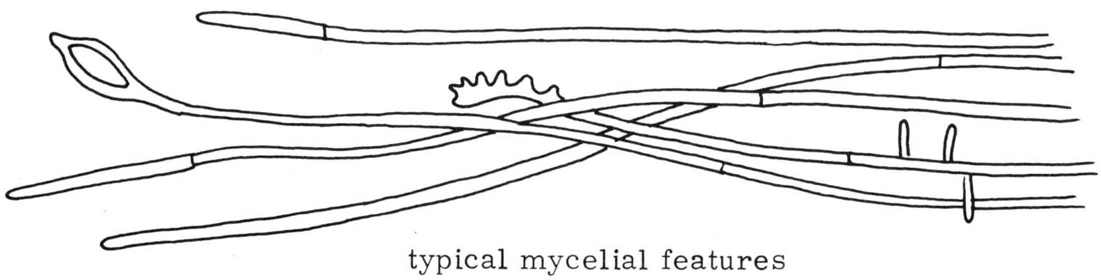

typical mycelial features

Microsporum audouinii - Cont.

Variants - Sporulating variants are a welcome interruption in the laboratory routine. Isolates with features of both M. canis and M. audouinii have been reported and have not been satisfactorily classified to date. Some strains, particularly an African form 'langeronii', develop more radial grooves and also a rose-tan color. The langeronii variant is perhaps slightly more pathogenic for the guinea pig, producing some fluorescent hairs. M. audouinii var. rivalieri is present in both Leopoldville, Republic of the Congo, and Miami, Florida, USA, to the extent of about 15 percent of M. audouinii strains isolated, and is only very rarely seen elsewhere. Variety rivalieri has a greyish white, much folded thallus, somewhat suggestive of T. schoenleinii, but tending to be more fluffy in the presence of yeast extract. A satin-like sheen is often seen on the surface of the thallus, the edge of which usually exhibits the appearance of coarse ground glass. The rivalieri variant is characterized microscopically by inflated and bulbous pectinate hyphae, and very occasionally macroaleuriospores of the M. audouinii type. The rivalieri variant grows rapidly. Like M. audouinii it does not become pleomorphic, but unlike typical M. audouinii the thallus quickly dies unless subcultured before it has reached the limits of the available agar surface, and it does not remain viable in the refrigerator.

Perfect State - Unknown. Strains tested against A. simii have been (+) mating type.

Special Media - Polished rice and potato dextrose agar are useful in separating M. audouinii from M. canis.* Addition of yeast extract to the medium may stimulate formation of pectinate hyphae and rarely macroaleuriospores in some strains of M. audouinii. Macroaleuriospores are sometimes obtained in soil-hair cultures. * var. rivalieri grows slightly on rice.

Critical Characteristics - (1) Appearance of the thallus, (2) Absence of macroaleuriospores (except in rare strains), (3) Terminal chlamydospores and pectinate hyphae, (4) Failure to grow on polished rice, (5) Macroaleuriospores when produced, (6) Lack of pathogenicity for the guinea pig.

References:

Zaias, N., Rebell, G., and Taplin, D., 1965. Microsporum rivalieri Vanbreuseghem Isolated from Tinea Capitis in Florida, Sabouraudia, 4, 201-204.

Whittle, C.H. and Gresham, G.A., 1970. Microsporum rivalieri Isolated from Tinea Capitis in East Anglia (England), Sabouraudia, 8, 65-71.

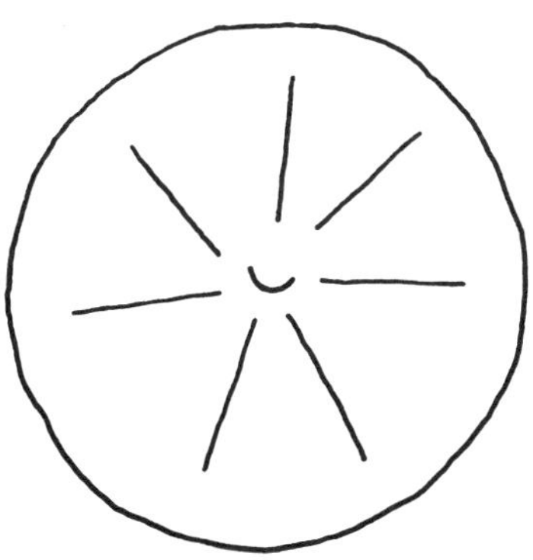

thallus with radial grooves

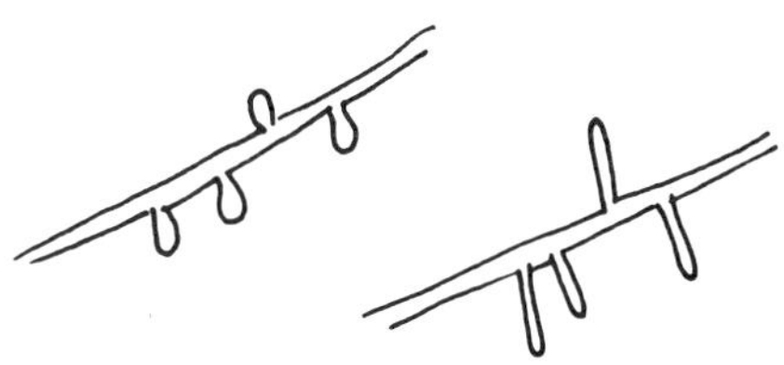

microaleuriospores

Microsporum audouinii - Cont.

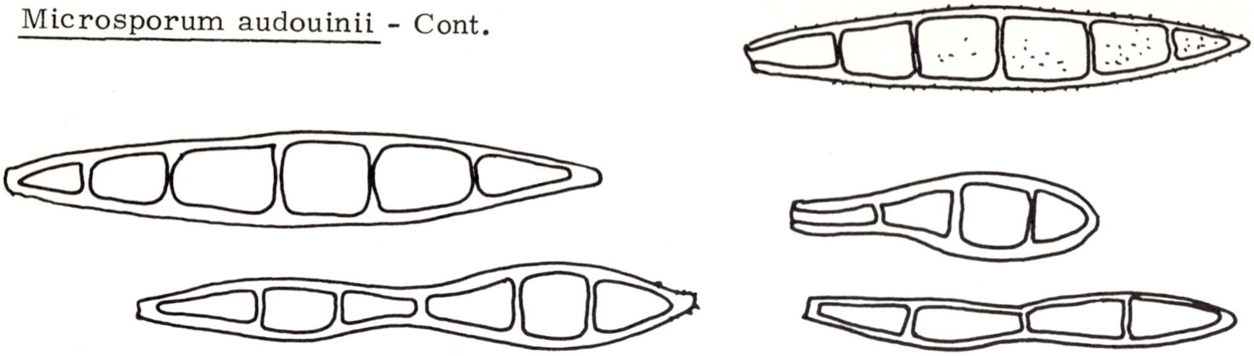

macroaleuriospores
of M. audouinii

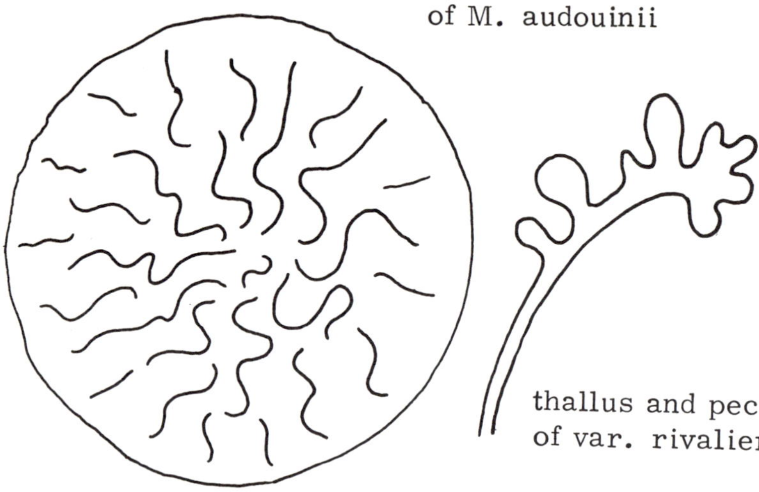

thallus and pectinate hypha
of var. rivalieri

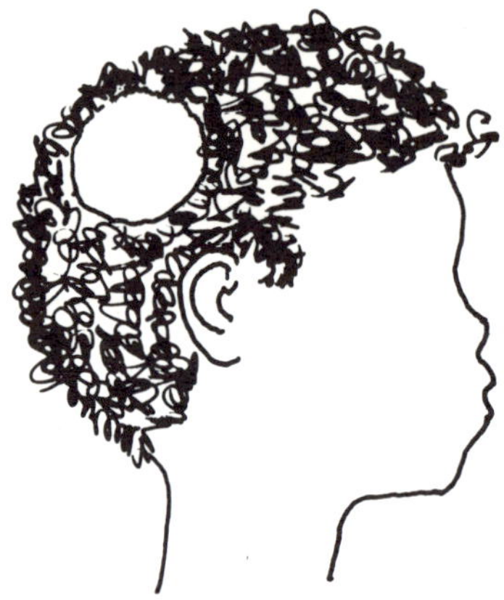

"grey patch" lesion typical of
of parasitic Microsporum
ringworm

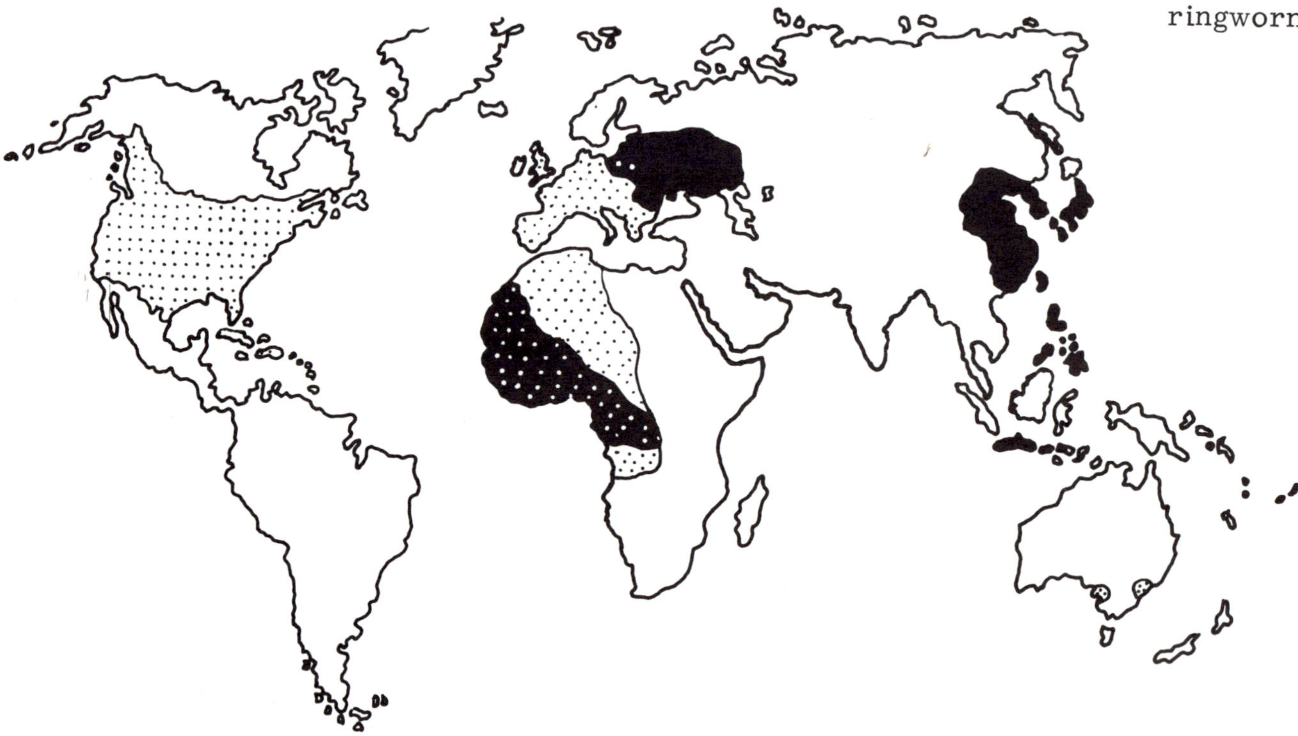

major distribution of epidemic fluorescent tinea capitis

M. audouinii ⬚ M. ferrugineum ■

Identification of <u>Microsporum ferrugineum</u>

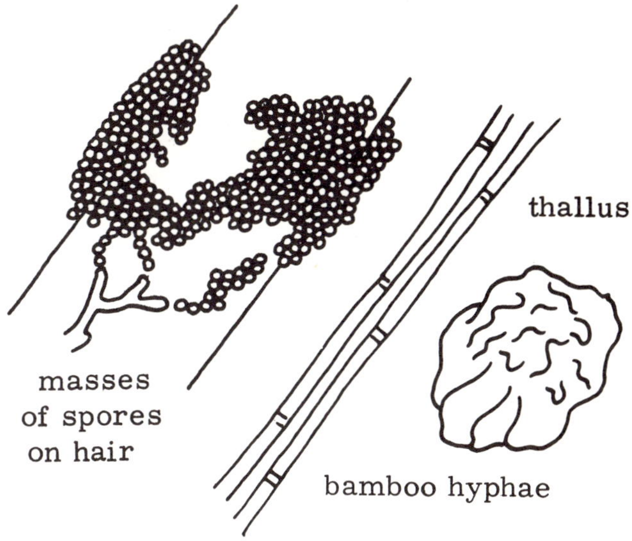

Invasion of Hair - Similar to M. canis; ectothrix, small spores in masses, hair usually fluorescent.

Clinical Disease - Primarily juvenile tinea capitis, usually non-inflammatory.

Epidemiology - Anthropophilic, epidemic tinea capitis.

Geographical Distribution - Asia, USSR, Eastern Europe, and Africa. A common species in Japan and Africa. Rare or unknown in the Western Hemisphere, except in Brazil where a single apparently endemic case has been reported. Endemic in the Balkans. Possibly increasing in Eastern Europe following relocation of Oriental peoples during World War II. Present in Hawaii. Reported as exclusive cause of fluorescent tinea capitis in Bulgaria and adjacent Romania and USSR. Map Page 18.

Appearance of Thallus - There are two forms: (1) glabrous, slow-growing, heaped-up and yellow to rust colored, as shown in Color Plate 1 which is the form prevalent in the Far East, and (2) more flat and leathery, spreading, and to some extent white and downy, which is the "album" form prevalent in the Balkans. Although one or the other form may predominate regionally, both are found throughout the geographic range of the species. M. ferrugineum has a marked tendency to develop sectors of different color intensity and is difficult to maintain in the laboratory in its pigmented form. Not viable in the refrigerator. May resemble M. canis, T. soudanense, or T. verrucosum var. ochraceum. Plate I.

Microscopic Morphology - Usually only sterile mycelia, which may be irregularly branched, fragmented, and clubbed. Sometimes with characteristic coarse, long, straight hyphae with prominant cross walls ("bamboo" hyphae). Macroaleuriospores most resembling those of M. canis and M. cookei have been reported in 5 of 23 African isolates grown on potato dextrose charcoal agar (freezing agar) and diluted Sabouraud's agar.

Variants - The two major varieties are described above under Morphology of Thallus. There is usually considerable variation in the form and color of the thallus, due in part to marked tendency to sector and become pleomorphic.

Special Nutritional Requirements - None reported.

Perfect State - Not known.

Special Media - May be differentiated from T. soudanense by light yellowish rather than dark brownish-red thallus on Lowenstein's medium* and possibly by urease activity. * See page 56.

Microsporum ferrugineum - Cont.

Critical Characteristics - (1) Appearance of thallus, (2) Type of hair invasion, (3) Does not require thiamine, (4) Geographical distribution, (5) Usual absence of macroaleuriospores.

References:

Vanbreuseghem, R., 1950. Étude de 136 souches de Trichophyton ferrugineum (Ota 1921) Langeron et Milochevitch 1930 et de sa varieté blanche, isolées au Congo Belge, Ann. Parasitol. Hum. et Comp., 25:485-492.

Vanbreuseghem, R., 1958. Mycoses of Man and Animals, transl. by J. Wilkinson, Sir Isaac Pitman and Sons, Ltd., London, pp. 104-105. Masson et Cie, Éditeurs, Paris.

Vanbreuseghem, R., 1966. Guide Pratique de Mycologie Médicale et Vétérinaire, Masson et Cie, Éditeurs, Paris.

Vanbreuseghem, R., DeVroly, C., and Takashio, M., 1970. Production of Macroconidia by Microsporum ferrugineum Ota 1922, Sabouraudia, 7:252-256.

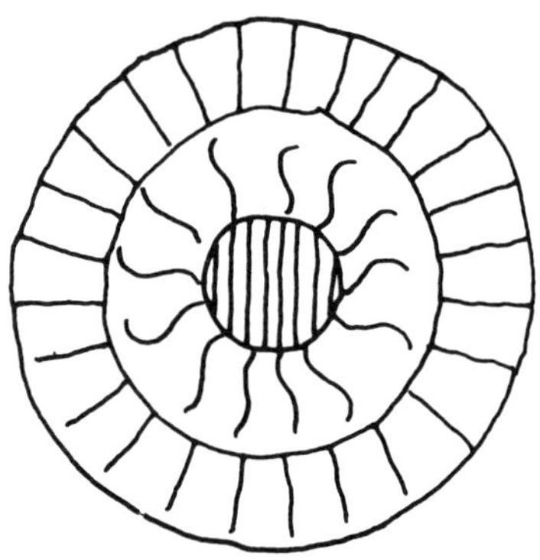

mature thallus of album form

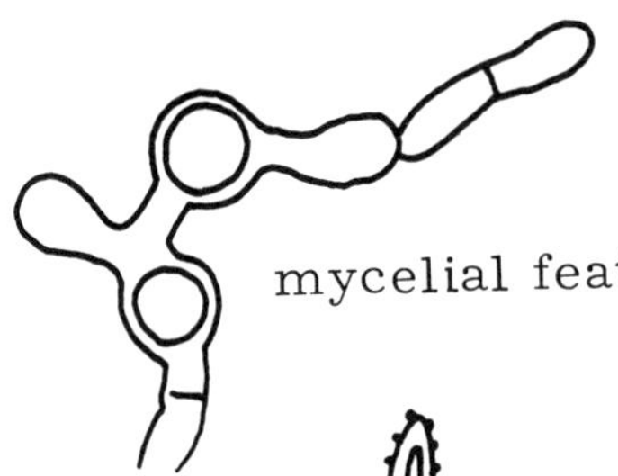

mycelial feature

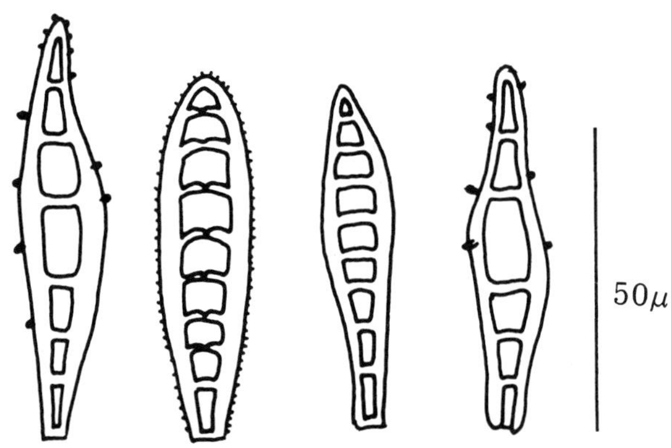

Macroaleuriospores of four African isolates of M. ferrugineum drawn the same size as photomicrographs on page 84 (700X as printed). The majority observed were somewhat smaller (40-50μ) (After Vanbreuseghem, DeVroly, and Takashio, 1970).

Identification of Trichophyton (Microsporum?) gallinae

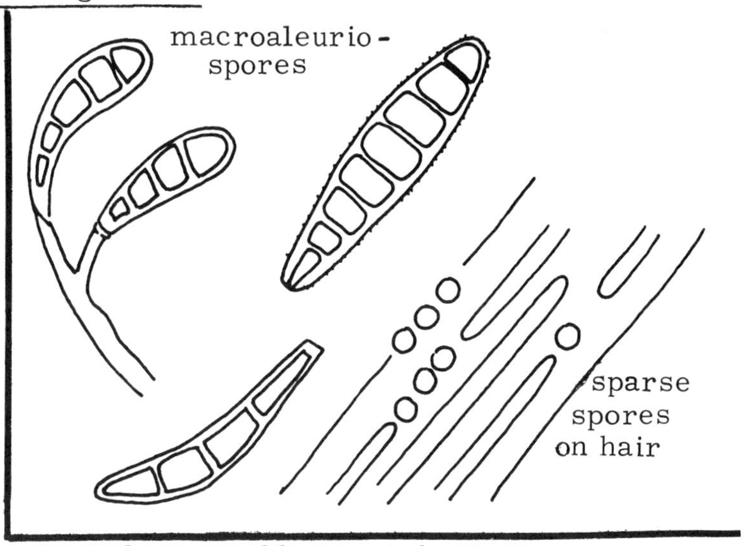

Note - On the basis of a recent report of rough-walled macroaleuriospores in an initially atypical isolate, we class this species as a Microsporum. However, since this manual is not a suitable place to publish changes in taxonomy, we have retained the name of this species as Trichophyton gallinae.

Invasion of Hair - Sparse ectothrix.

Clinical Disease - Scalp ringworm and possible tinea corporis. Only two authenticated cases of human infection are known, both in children.

Epidemiology - The cause of ringworm in chickens and other fowl, affecting the comb and wattles producing "white comb" lesions, and also the feather parts. See also T. simii.

Geographical Distribution - World-wide.

Appearance of Thallus - A slightly downy or satiny white thallus turning pink and buff with age and usually producing a characteristic pigment, initially yellow but becoming strawberry-red which diffuses into the agar. Sporulating strain isolated from Philippine monkey resembled M. gypseum and produced yellow-red pigment when first isolated. Plate II.

Microscopic Morphology - Macroaleuriospores more or less abundant, the largest of which tend to be blunt-tipped and slipper shape in profile, with 5 to 6 cells or more, usually smooth, but sometimes slightly echinulate, particularly on soil-extract agar. A distinctive feature is the frequent presence of curved and proximally tapered macroaleuriospores, and the attachment of the macroaleuriospores to toothed, pectinate, or leaf-like hyphae. Club-shaped or pear-shaped microaleuriospores in moderate numbers.

Special Nutritional Requirements - None known.

Variants - Fresh isolates may be suggestive of M. gypseum and initially fail to produce strawberry pigment. Pleomorphic colonies become fluffy and lose the characteristic pigment production.

Perfect State - Not reported.

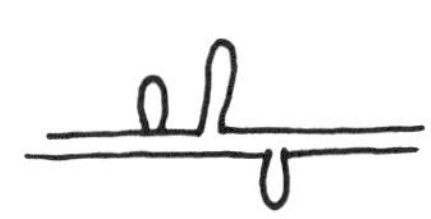

microaleuriospores

Trichophyton (Microsporum?) gallinae - Cont.

Special Media - Not required. Confusion with the histidine-requiring T. megninii previously existed, but the two species clearly differ on several counts.

Critical Characteristics - (1) Appearance of thallus and diffusing pigment, (2) Microscopic morphology, (3) Characteristic lesions in chickens.

References:

Georg, L.K., 1952. Cultural and Nutritional Studies of Trichophyton gallinae and Trichophyton megninii, Mycologia 44:470-492.

Torres, G. and Georg, L.K., 1956. A Human Case of Trichophyton gallinae Infection. Disease Contracted from Chickens, Arch. Dermat., 74: 191-197.

Gordon, M.A. and Little, G.N., 1968. Trichophyton (Microsporum?) gallinae Ringworm in a Monkey, Sabouraudia, 6:207-212.

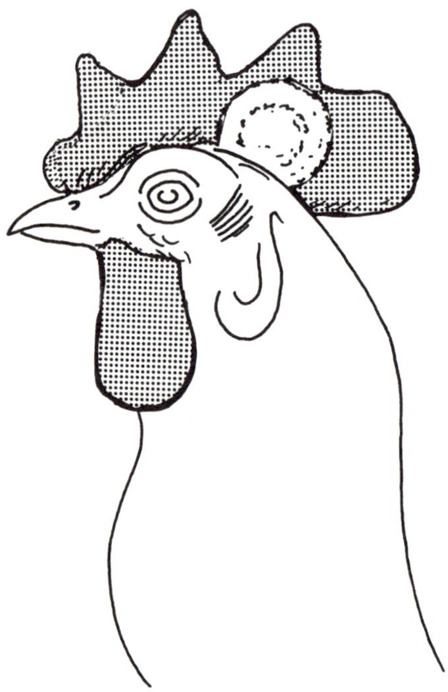

lesion of T. (M?) gallinae

MICROSPORUM SPECIES COMMON IN VETERINARY MEDICINE

M. canis (cats, dogs, horses, primates) commonly transmitted to man.

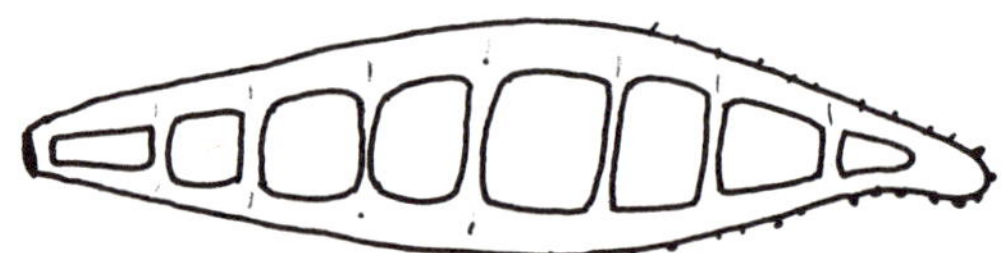

13

M. gypseum (geophilic) infects man and animals.

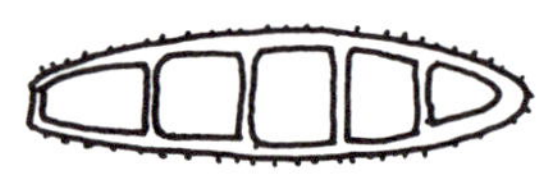

23

T.(M?) gallinae (gallinaceous birds) rarely transmitted to man.

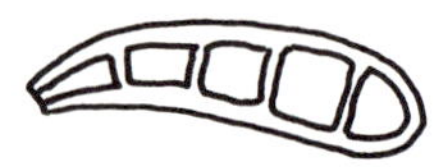

21

M. canis obesum forms (principally horses, primates and man).

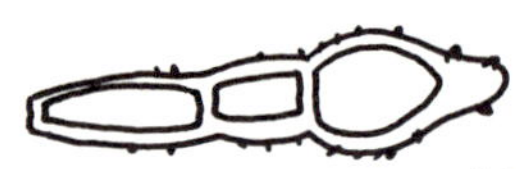

13

M. audouinii (common in man) rarely transmitted to dogs.

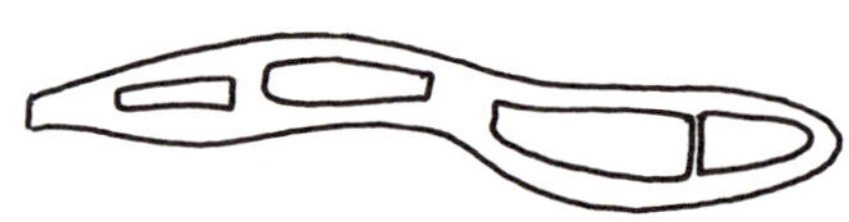

16

M. nanum (pigs) occasionally transmitted to man.

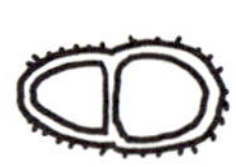

26

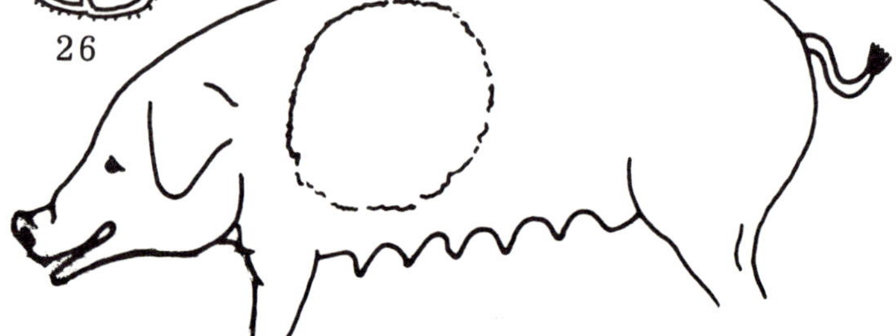

lesion of M. nanum

Identification of Microsporum gypseum

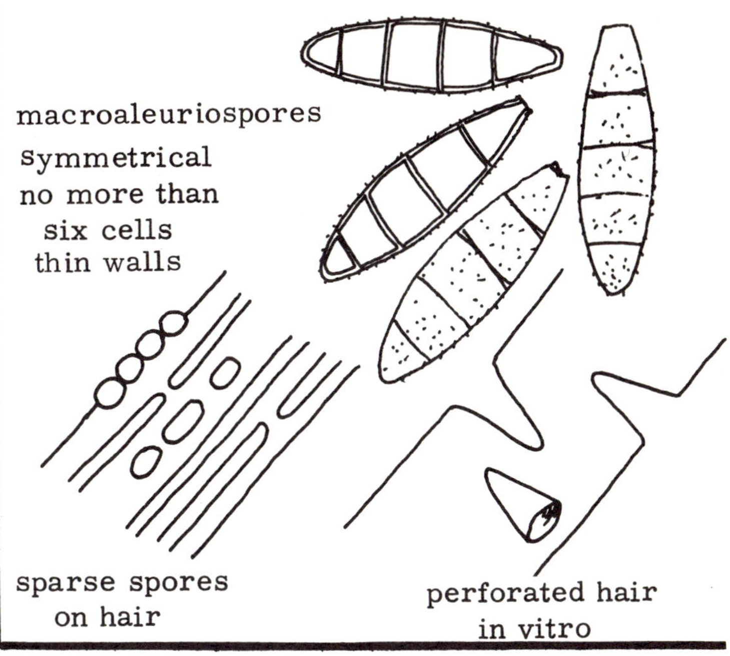

Invasion of Hair - Sporulation is mainly ectothrix but sparse and in chains. Fluorescence of hair, if any, is dull. Perforates hair in vitro.

Clinical Disease - Tinea corporis and tinea capitis. Lesions usually single or few, usually inflammatory, impetiginous, and sometimes bullous, with rapid course and resolution. May produce favus-like crusts.

Epidemiology - Common in soil, especially in rich garden soils. Infections in man occasional, in children and other persons in contact with soil. Infections occur in a large variety of animals. See page 22.

Geographical Distribution - World-wide.

Appearance of Thallus - A characteristic rapidly spreading thallus, spreading texture of chamois, rich cinnamon-buff, due to multitudes of macroaleuriospores. Quickly develops diffuse pleomorphism. Plates I and IV.

Microscopic Morphology - Macroaleuriospores in enormous numbers, symmetrical, ellipsoidal structures with the shape of cucumber pickles. They have rough or echinulate surfaces and are relatively thin-walled with up to six compartments. Club-shaped microaleuriospores may be present, but are not diagnostic.

Special Nutritional Requirements - None reported.

Variants - There are two known species of Nannizzia which are recognized as distinct in their perfect state, but which are difficult to separate in their conidial forms, and are therefore included under the name of M. gypseum. A third species, M. fulvum, is more easily distinguished and is described separately (page 25). Strains belonging to the species Nannizzia gypsea produce more spreading and heavily powdery thalli, with brighter surface color, and often veins of deeper pigment beneath. Macroaleuriospores tend to be somewhat more plump. A red pigmented form (not M. cookei) is sometimes isolated from soil and small mammals. Strains belonging to Nannizzia incurvata may be yellow or reddish beneath. A reddish brown mutant of N. gypsea isolated from soil produced smooth macroaleuriospores. A rather similar mutant of N. gypsea, described as var. vinosum, isolated from a clinical lesion produces few macroaleuriospores and a sparsely silky thallus, suggestive of M. canis but with a reddish brown surface and undersurface. The initial outgrowth from the clinical specimen was subsurface and brilliant yellow, resembling that of some isolates of the sulfureum variety of T. tonsurans.

Microsporum gypseum - Cont.

Perfect State - Various strains of M. gypseum are imperfect states of at least two species, Nannizzia incurvata and Nannizzia gypsea (both heterothallic). Both are frequently isolated from clinical lesions. Less commonly the mated ascigerous forms may be isolated from ringworm lesions.

Special Media - None required.

Critical Characteristics - (1) Characteristic macroaleuriospores, (2) Thallus form, (3) To identify with N. incurvata or N. gypsea, ability to form asci with cultures grown from single ascospores of these species.

References:

Stockdale, P. M., 1963. The Microsporum gypseum Complex (Nannizzia incurvata Stockd., N. gypsea (Nann.) comb. nov., N. fulva sp. nov., Sabouraudia, 3:114-126.

Gordon, M. A. and Lusick, L. A., 1965. An Unusual Variant of M. gypseum (Nannizzia gypsea), Arch. Derm., 91:558-562.

Varsovsky, E., Weitzman, I., and Reca, M. E., 1966. A Smooth-Walled Mutant of Nannizzia gypsea (Nann.) Stockd. Isolated from Soil, Sabouraudia, 4:242-243.

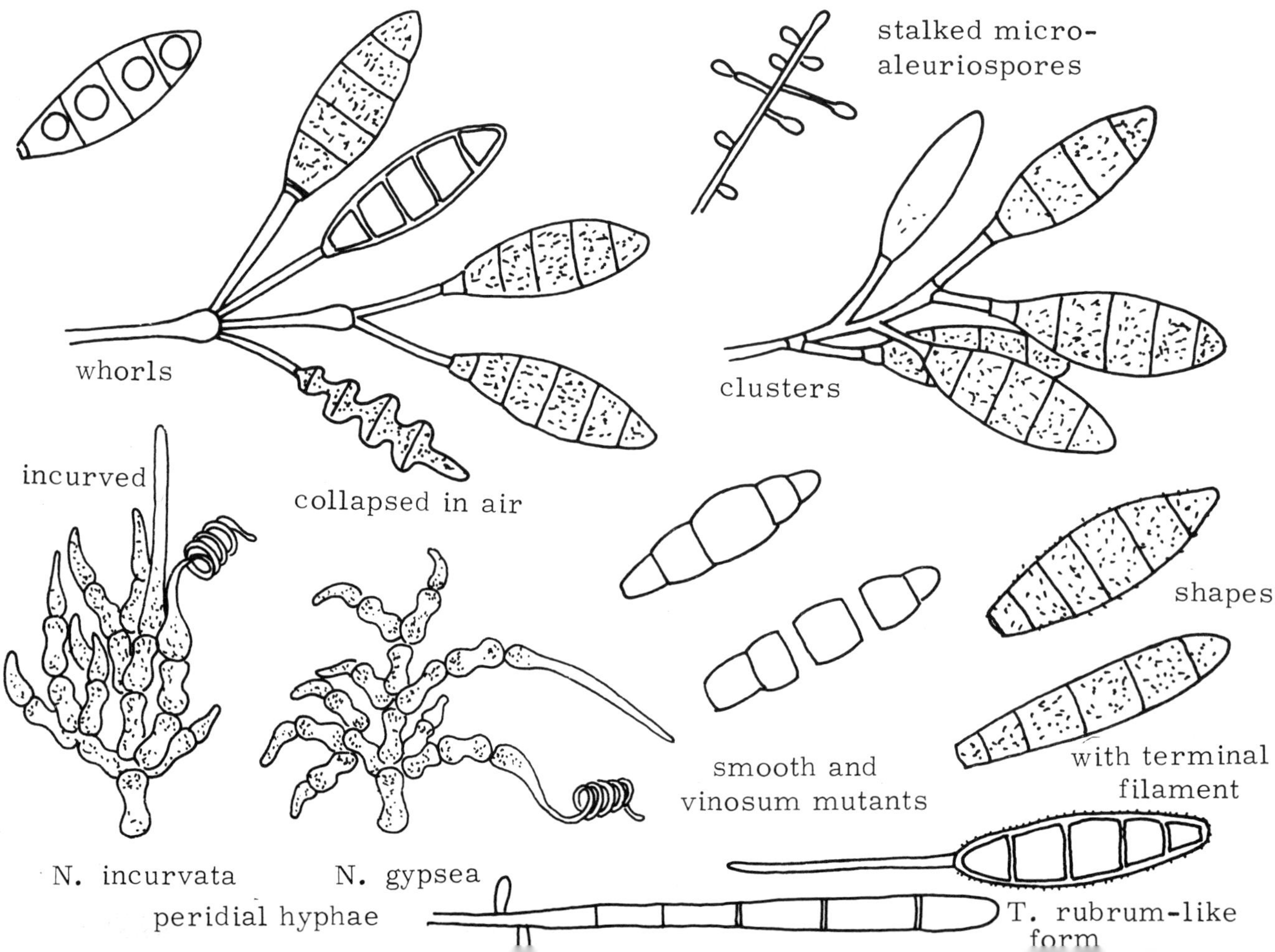

Identification of Microsporum fulvum

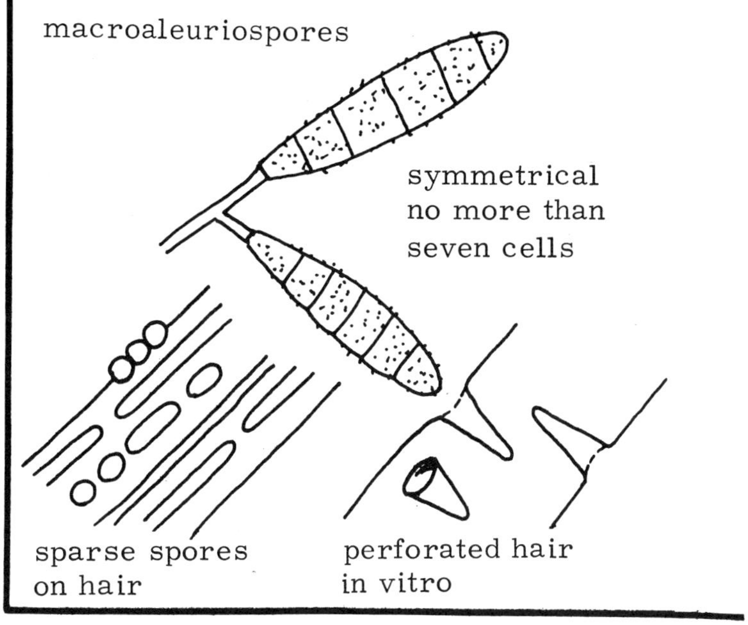

Invasion of Hair - Sparse ectothrix, similar to M. gypseum. Perforates hair in vitro.

Clinical Disease - Similar to M. gypseum but less common and usually not separated from it in previous literature. Possibly less pathogenic than M. gypseum.

Epidemiology - Present in soil. Occasional infections in man and animals.

Geographical Distribution - World-wide.

Appearance of Thallus - A rapidly growing, flat thallus with a dense downy to floccose chamois-like surface, tawny buff to pink buff in color, frequently with a fluffy white advancing edge. Undersurface of colony may be dark red. Plate I.

Microscopic Morphology - Large numbers of macroaleuriospores which closely resemble those of M. gypseum, but are longer and more clavate or bullet-shaped, frequently lateral and not conspicuously clustered. Spiral hyphae may be numerous and branched.

Special Nutritional Requirements - None reported.

Variants - Previously grouped as a variety of M. gypseum now separated. Most isolates can probably be identified by morphology in culture. See also M. boullardii.

Perfect State - Nannizzia fulva (heterothallic). Peridial hyphae most resemble those of M. gypsea.

Special Media - None required.

Critical Characteristics - (1) Characteristic macroaleuriospores, (2) Form of thallus, (3) Ascospores with tester strains of Nannizzia fulva.

References:

Stockdale, P. M., 1963. The Microsporum gypseum complex (Nannizzia incurvata Stockd., N. gypsea (Nann.) comb. nov., N. fulva sp. nov.), Sabouraudia, 3:114-126.

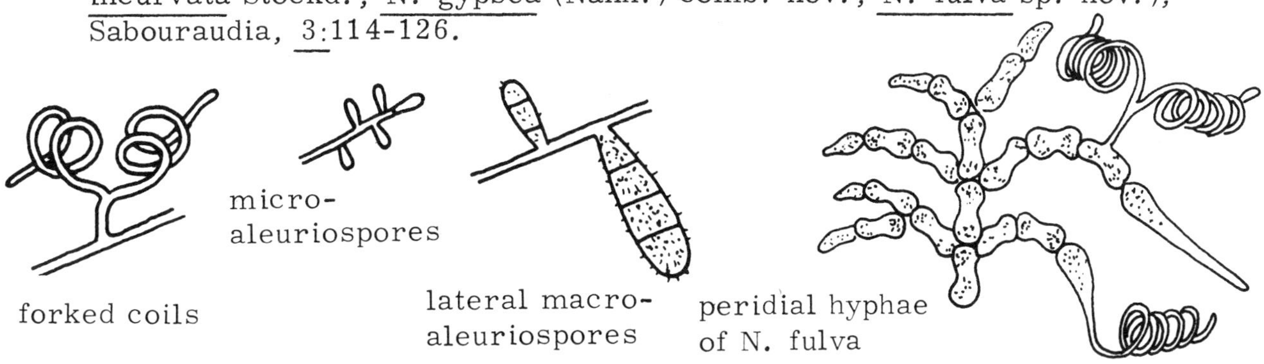

Identification of Microsporum nanum

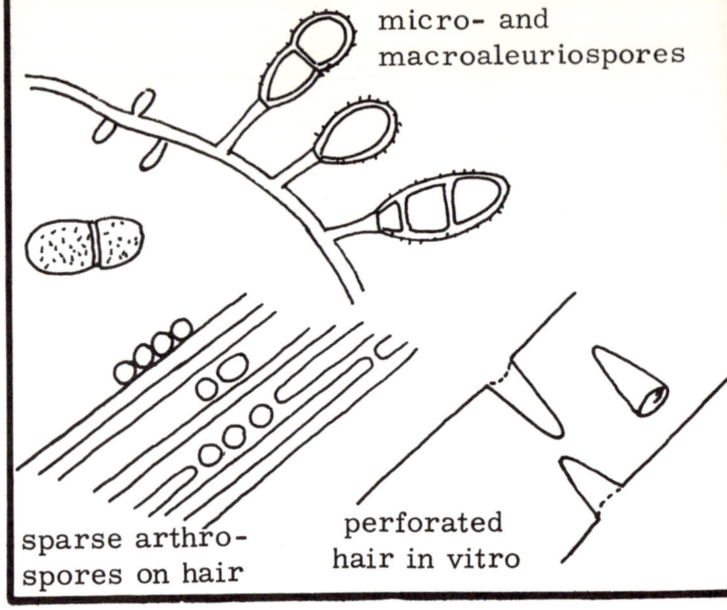

Invasion of Hair - Sparse ectothrix, similar to M. gypseum. Perforates hair in vitro.

Clinical Disease - A rare cause of tinea corporis and tinea capitis in man, similar to the more common M. gypseum. In pig, transient inflammatory ringworm in piglets, chronic, slowly spreading brownish circular lesions in adult pigs, lesions frequently behind the ears.

Epidemiology - The principle cause of ringworm in pigs. However, also present in soil in pigyards. Infections in man usually contacted directly from pig or fomites. See page 22.

Geographical Distribution - World-wide.

Appearance of Thallus - A thin spreading thallus with more or less of a powdery, dark buff surface due to the presence of macroaleuriospores. Undersurface of thallus frequently reddish brown. Plate I.

Microscopic Morphology - Characteristic rough-walled macroaleuriospores are egg-shaped to ellipsoidal ovate and consist of only one to three cells (rarely four). Relatively thin walls, suggesting M. gypseum. Microaleuriospores clavate, not specific for the species, but separate it from Chrysosporium species having large egg-shaped aleuriospores which can be confused with M. nanum macroaleuriospores.

Special Nutritional Requirements - None reported.

Variants - A reddish brown pigment usually develops under thallus.

Perfect State - Nannizzia obtusa (heterothallic). See illustration page 28.

Special Media - Not required.

Critical Characteristics - (1) Macro- and microaleuriospores, (2) Ascospores with tester strains of N. obtusa.

References:

Dawson, C.O. and Gentles, J.C., 1961. The Perfect States of Keratinomyces ajelloi Vanbreuseghem, Trichophyton terrestre Durie and Frey and Microsporum nanum Fuentes, Sabouraudia, 1:49-57.

Ajello, L., Varsovosky, E., Ginther, O.J. and Bubash, G., 1964. The Natural History of Microsporum nanum, Mycologia, 56:873-884.

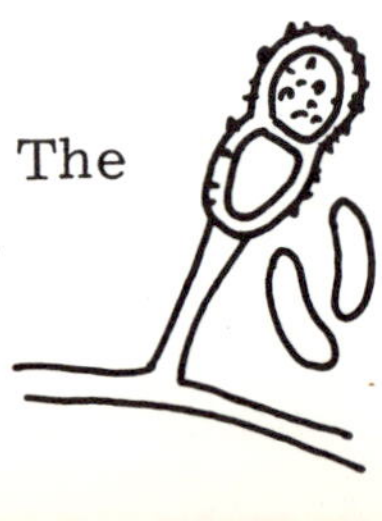

Chlamydospores and conidia of Fusarium, may be mistaken for M. nanum.

Identification of Microsporum persicolor

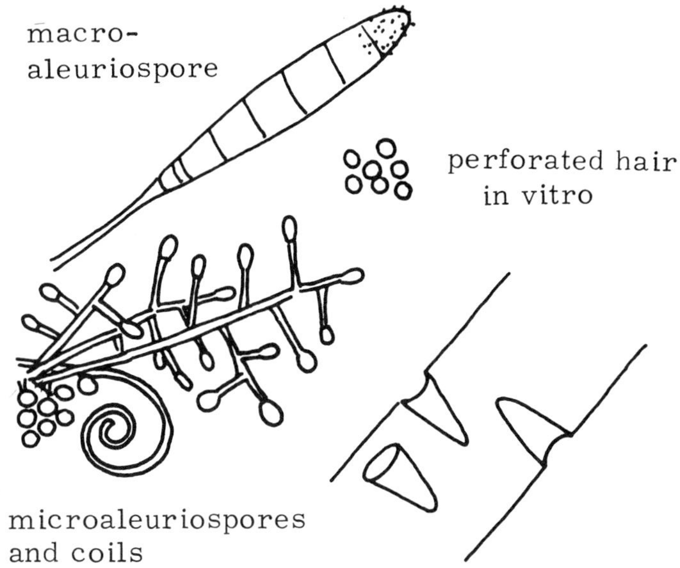

Invasion of Hair - Apparently does not parasitize hair. Perforates hair in vitro.

Clinical Disease - An uncommon cause of sporadic tinea corporis in Europe.

Epidemiology - Associated predominantly with the Bank Vole, Clethrionomys glareolus, on which it grows on the tail which may have scaling lesions. Also isolated from the fur of Bank Voles, Field Voles, Microtus agrestis, and others of these mice and other small mammals in the absence of lesions. Not isolated from the soil.

Geographical Distribution - Apparently restricted to the natural range of Bank and Field Voles (Europe and The British Isles) where it has been known as an occasional cause of tinea corporis since the time of Sabouraud (1910).

Appearance of Thallus - Rapidly growing, flat, fluffy, to densely powdery or suede-like, frequently with a fringed margin and surface color pale yellowish buff to pinkish buff with the undersurface various shades of ochre. Especially on sugar free media the thallus surface and undersurface characteristically develops rosy to deep wine tints and marginal zones which serve to distinguish M. persicolor from T. mentagrophytes. Plate IV.

Microscopic Morphology - Most suggestive of T. mentagrophytes, with large clusters of spherical or club-shaped microaleuriospores, rather coarse coils, and scattered, narrow, spindle-shaped or club-shaped, thin-walled, predominantly six celled macroaleuriospores which may be echinulate at the tip. Fresh isolates may be distinguished by the rapid production of very large numbers of spiral hyphae and macroaleuriospores. Differing from T. mentagrophytes by having microaleuriospores rather predominantly stalked and club-shaped when immature as in the M. gypseum complex.

Special Nutritional Requirements - None. Probably grows better than T. mentagrophytes on inorganic nitrogen.

Variants - A particularly deeply pigmented strain has been isolated from a bat (Pipistrellus sp.). M. persicolor was for many years mistakenly considered to be a rare variant of T. mentagrophytes by American workers.

Perfect State - Nannizzia persicolor (heterothallic).

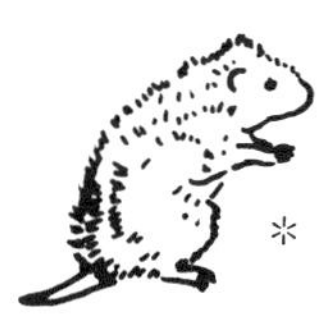

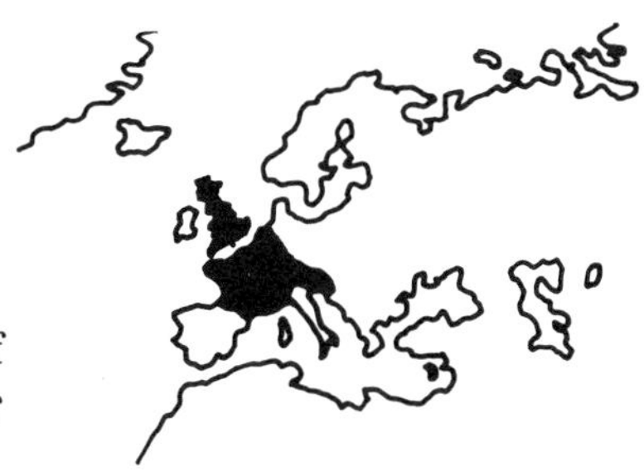

distribution of M. persicolor

* English and Southern, 1967. Sabouraudia 5:302-309.

Microsporum persicolor - Cont.

Special Media - Distinctive pink-wine colors develop on sugar-free peptone agar. Formation of macroaleuriospores favored by alkaline pH. The rough surface of the macroaleuriospores is most evident on soil-hair substrates.

Critical Characteristics - (1) Microscopic features, (2) Appearance of thallus on sugar-free medium, (3) Ascospores with tester strain of N. persicolor, (4) Not yet reported outside of Europe and British Isles.

References:

Stockdale, P. M., 1967. Nannizzia persicolor sp. nov., The Perfect State of Trichophyton persicolor, Sabouraudia 5:355-359.

English, M. P., 1966. Trichophyton persicolor Infections in the Field Vole and Pipestrelle Bat, Sabouraudia 4:219-222.

Vanbreuseghem, R., 1949. Contribution à la connaissance de Ctenomyces persicolor. Rapport d'un cas personnel. Ann. Parasit. hum. comp. 24, 124.

peridial hyphae of four species of Nannizzia

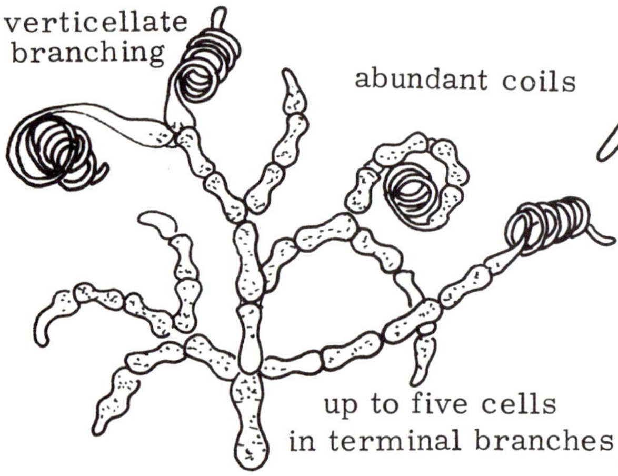

N. persicolor

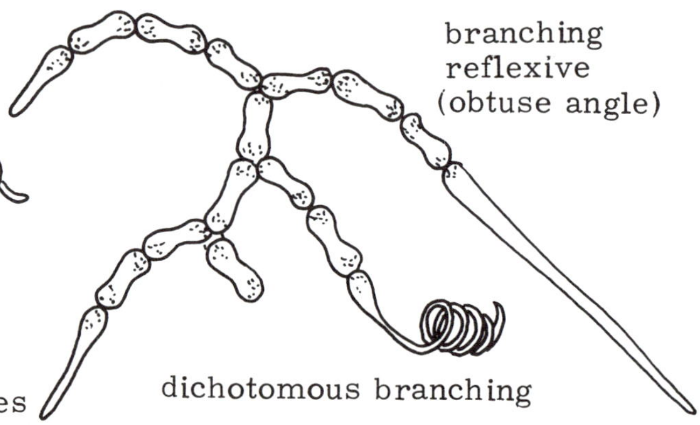

26 N. obtusa

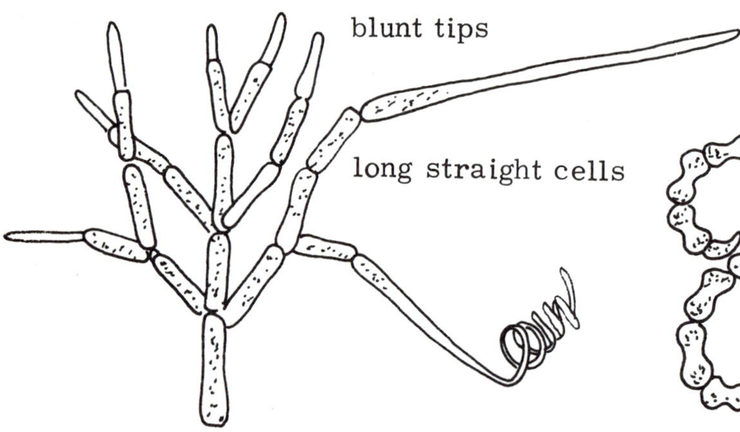

29 N. cajetani

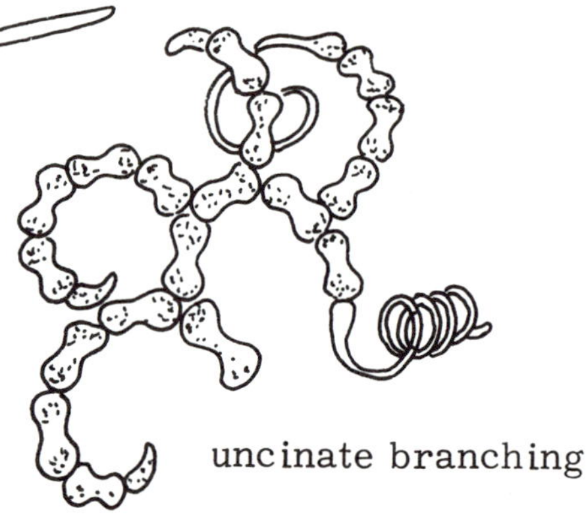

30 N. grubyia

Identification of Microsporum cookei

macroaleuriospores

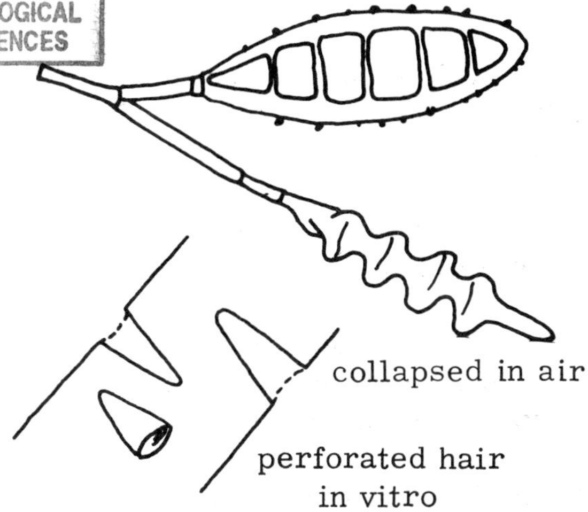

Invasion of Hair - Not known to invade hair. Perforates hair in vitro.

Clinical Disease - Not certainly known to cause infections in man or lesions in animals. Infection reported in dog and eczematous lesions in man.

Epidemiology - A geophilic species isolated from soil and the hair of small mammals.

Geographical Distribution - World-wide.

Appearance of Thallus - A coarse spreading thallus usually with a characteristic deep grape-red pigment. Surface usually becomes more or less powdery and yellowish or greenish buff to dark brown due to production of macroaleuriospores. Plate I.

Microscopic Morphology - Oval echinulate macroaleuriospores with thick to markedly thick walls. Thick walls serve to distinguish species from red isolates of M. gypseum. Microaleuriospores usually abundant and obovoid but not safely diagnostic.

Special Nutritional Requirements - None reported.

Variants - There is a considerable range of macroaleuriospore types. An isolate with a peculiar membrane around the macroaleuriospores has been reported.

Perfect State - Nannizzia cajetani (heterothallic). Isolates which fail to mate with N. cajetani are suspected of being other as yet undescribed species with an M. cookei conidial state. See illustration page 28.

Special Media - Not required.

Critical Characteristics - (1) Macroaleuriospores, (2) Characteristics of thallus, (3) Ascospores with tester strains of N. cajetani.

References:

Ajello, L., 1959. A New Microsporum and Its Occurrence on Man and Animals, Mycologia, 51:69-76.

Ajello, L., 1961. The Ascigerous State of Microsporum cookei, Sabouraudia, 1:173-177.

Lundell, E., 1965. Microsporum cookei Ajello, An Eczematous Skin Lesion, Mykosen, 12:123-126.

Mariat, F. and Tapia, G., 1966. Observations sur une souche de Microsporum cookei parasite du Cynocephale (Papio papio), Sabouraudia, 5:43-45.

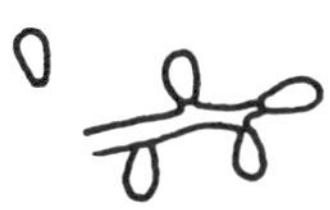

microaleuriospores

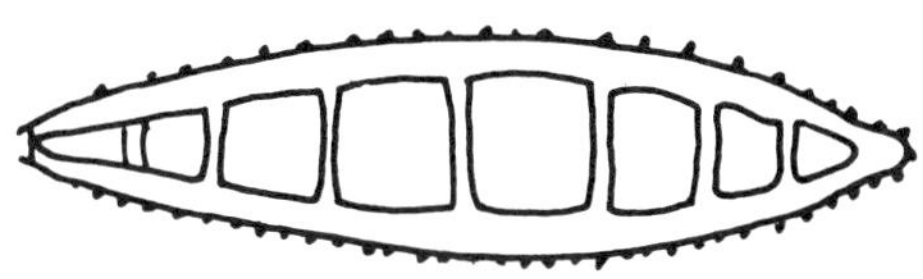

macroaleuriospore with terminal knob

Identification of Microsporum vanbreuseghemii

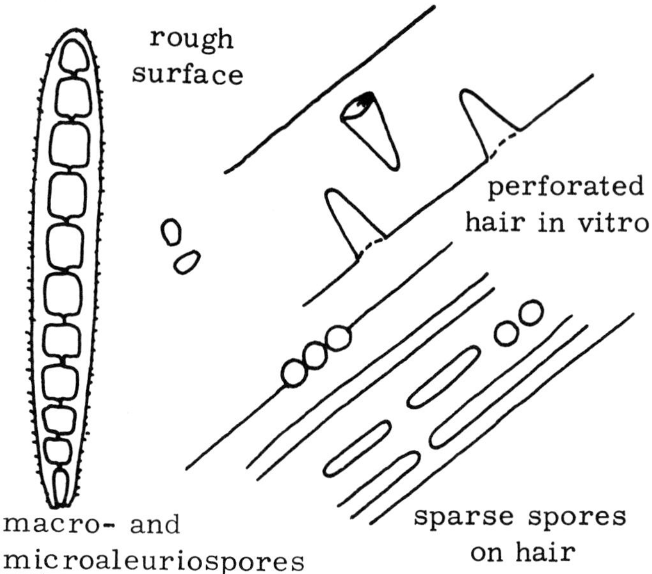

Invasion of Hair - Sparse chains of large ectothrix spores on hair. Not fluorescent. Perforates hair in vitro.

Clinical Disease - Rare cause of ringworm in man and animals.

Epidemiology - Has been isolated from soil. Capable of producing occasional infections in man and animals.

Geographical Distribution - So far isolated reports from the United States, Russia, India, and Africa.

Appearance of Thallus - A rapidly spreading somewhat cottony fluffy thallus which develops a lavender-pink to buff powdery surface, due to the aleuriospores. Undersurface of colonies colorless or yellow. Thallus of M. racemosum of the M. gypseum complex is similar, but produces wine-red to grape-purple color beneath. Plate I.

Microscopic Morphology - Long, tapered, many-celled macroaleuriospores with moderately thick walls, usually a rough surface, and frequently 8 or more cells. The echinulate surface and longer more slender pedicles serve to distinguish the mature macroaleuriospores from those of T. ajelloi, and walls thicker than septa and larger numbers of cells from those of M. racemosum and M. praecox. Microaleuriospores are usually obovoid, but not diagnostic.

Special Nutritional Requirements - None reported.

Variants - More or less fluffy forms are isolated and pleomorphism occurs readily.

Perfect State - Nannizzia grubyia (heterothallic). See illustration pages page 28 and 31.

Special Media - Not required.

Critical Characteristics - (1) Capacity to mate and produce ascospores with tester strains of N. grubyia, (2) Macroaleuriospores with thickened and roughened walls (see T. ajelloi, M. racemosum, and M. praecox), (3) Appearance of thallus, (4) Morphology of perfect state.

References:

Georg, L.K., Ajello, L., Friedman, L. and Brinkman, S.A., 1962. A New Species of Microsporum Pathogenic to Man and Animals, Sabouraudia 1:189-196.

Identification of Trichophyton ajelloi

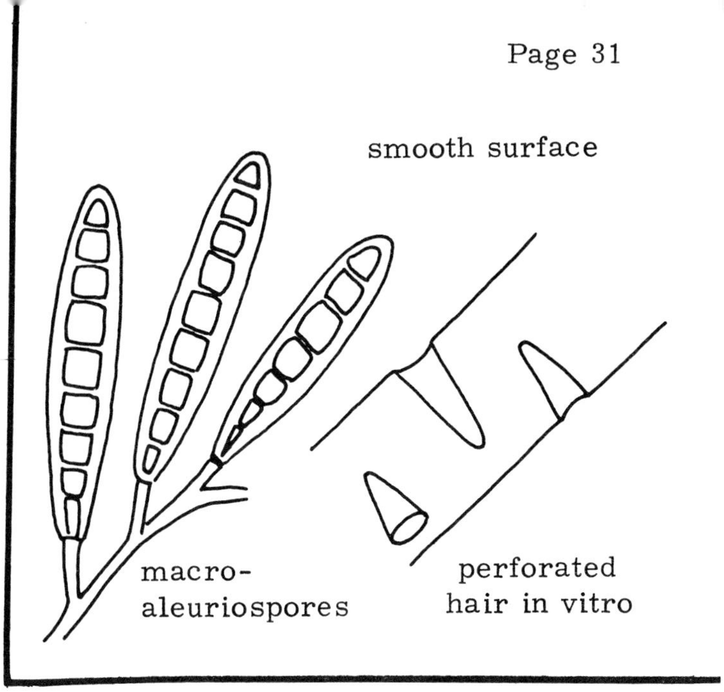

Invasion of Hair - Not known. Perforates hair in vitro.

Clinical Disease - Infections in man and animals doubtful. A possible vesicular lesion of the hand has been reported.

Epidemiology - Dermatophyte in soil.

Geographical Distribution - World-wide.

Appearance of Thallus - A relatively non-fluffy thallus with more or less of a powdery surface of rich orange buff to tan color. Usually produces a blackish purple pigment in the medium. Plate IV.

Microscopic Morphology - Powdery surface due to presence of usually large numbers of long, cigar shaped, many-celled macroaleuriospores, with moderately thick walls and smooth surfaces. Superficially may suggest E. floccosum (see E. floccosum). Microaleuriospores may be present, but are usually absent.

Special Nutritional Requirements - None reported.

Variants - Strains and mutants lacking purple-black undercolor occur. Pleomorphism in T. ajelloi occurs readily. A form with small macroaleuriospores has been described as T. ajelloi var. nana (see also T. longifusus).

Perfect State - Arthroderma uncinatum (heterothallic), has curved rough peridial hyphae with dumbbell-shaped cells. Sexuality has been recently demonstrated to be independent of production of black pigment. T. ajelloi var. nana does not produce ascospores with A. uncinatum and therefore may not be conspecific.

Special Media - Perfect state obtained from mating of strains on soil baited with horse hair.

Critical Characteristics - (1) Characteristic smooth walled macroaleuriospores, (2) Buff powdery surface of thallus, (3) Purple-black pigment, (4) Capacity to produce ascospores with tester strain of A. uncinatum (except in variety nana).

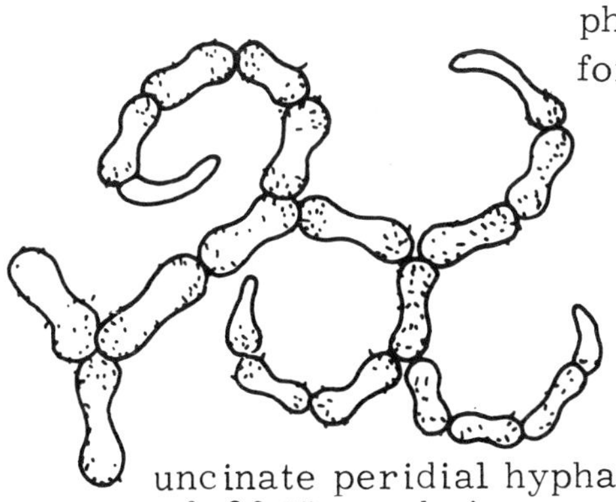

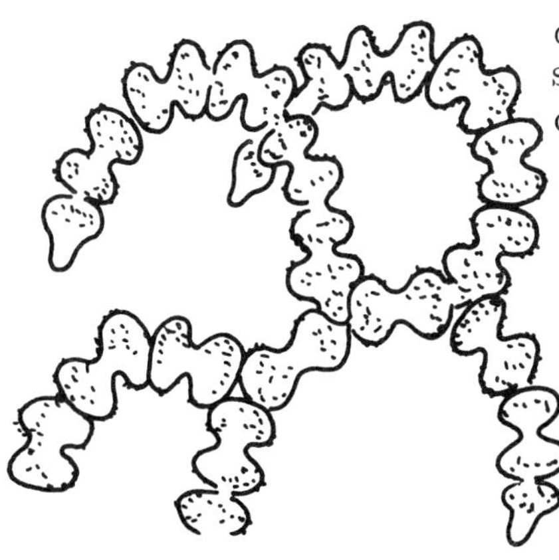

Trichophyton ajelloi - Cont.

References:

Georg, L.K., Kaplan, W., Ajello, L., Williamson, W.M. and Tilden, E.B., 1959. The Parasitic Nature of the Soil Fungus Keratinomyces ajelloi, J. Invest. Dermat., 32:539-544.

Dawson, C.O. and Gentles, J.C., 1961. The Perfect States of Keratinomyces ajelloi Vanbreuseghem; Trichophyton terrestre Durie & Frey and Microsporum nanum, Fuentes, Sabouraudia, 1:49-57.

Hejtmanek, M. and Kunert, J., 1966. A Dwarf Form of Keratinomyces ajelloi, Sabouraudia 4:3-5.

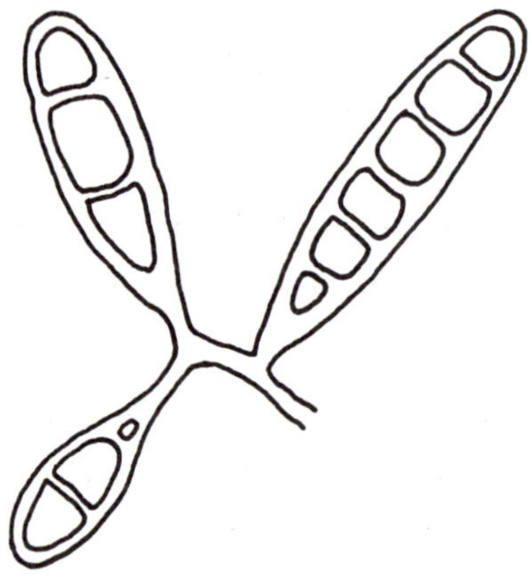

macroaleuriospores of T. ajelloi resembling Epidermophyton

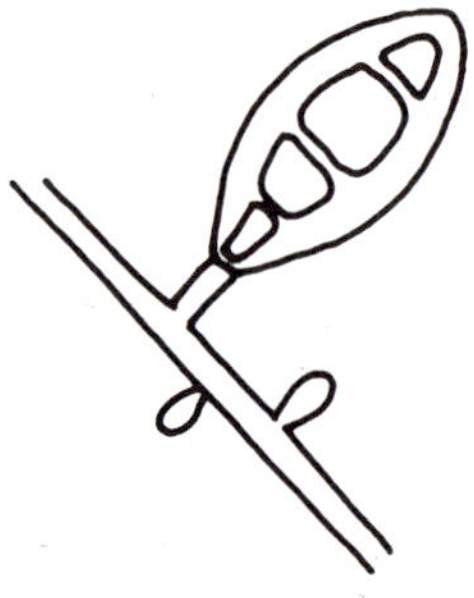

T. ajelloi var. nana

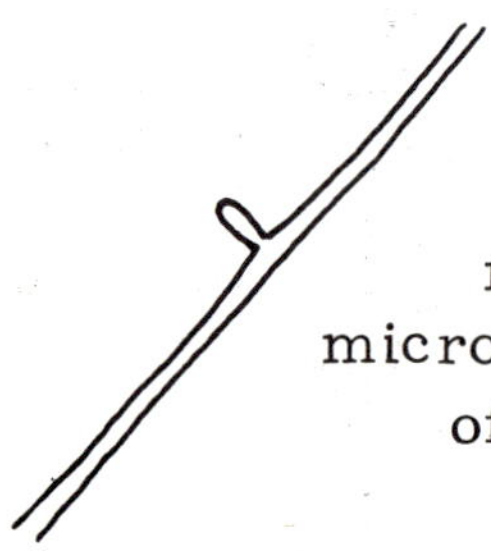

rare microaleuriospores of T. ajelloi

DERMATOPHYTES COMMONLY ISOLATED FROM SOIL

Widespread Species

M. gypseum (frequently pathogenic for man and animals).

T. ajelloi (doubtful infection in man and animals).

T. terrestre complex (no infections in man or animals).

Chrysosporium spp. and Arthroderma spp. (no infections reported in man and animals).

M. cookei (rare infections in man and animals).

Less Common Species and Recently Described Species

Other geophilic Microsporum spp. (rarely pathogenic for man and animals).

T. georgiae - (not pathogenic).

T. gloriae - (not pathogenic).

T. vanbreuseghemii - (rare infections in man and animals).

Present Locally in Soil

M. nanum (pigyards) commonly infects pigs.

T. simii (India) frequently infects man and animals.

T. mentagrophytes (small animal habitats) frequently infects man and animals.

Identification of Trichophyton terrestre

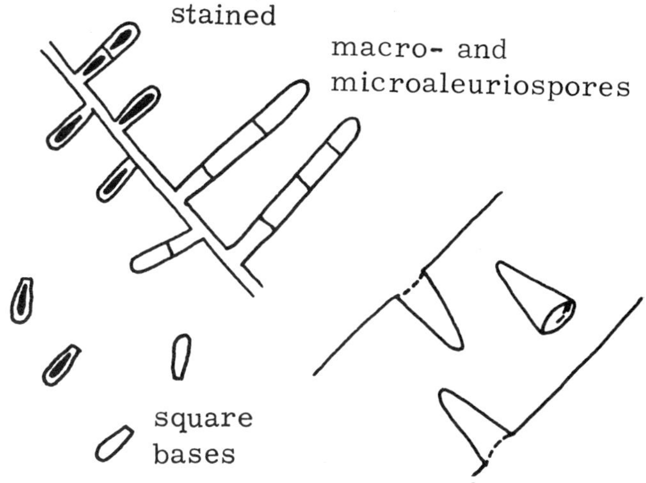

Invasion of Hair - Not known. Perforates hair in vitro.

Clinical Disease - Not known to cause infections in man or lesions in animals.

Epidemiology - Geophilic species isolated from the soil (particularly poor, alkaline and arid soils), and from the hair of small mammals. May occur as contaminant on human skin.

Geographical Distribution - World-wide.

Appearance of Thallus - A buff to yellow, powdery to granular thallus which may resemble T. mentagrophytes. However, the surface color may range from white to cream, yellow, or greenish yellow. Yellow or reddish pigment may be present under the thallus. Plate II.

Microscopic Morphology - Characteristic large clavate or pedicled microaleuriospores which usually exhibit transition forms to more or less abundant, lateral macroaleuriospores. The aleuriospores sometimes stain more intensely than hyphae with cotton blue, and have a prominant attachment scar. Spiral coils may be seen but are not diagnostic. The presence of well developed lateral macroaleuriospores (4-8 cells) separates the present species from some undescribed fungi with a T. terrestre-like microscopic appearance. Other species which may resemble T. terrestre are T. thuringiense, A. multifidum, T. longifusus, and T. gloriae.

Special Nutritional Requirements - None reported.

Variants - A slower growing deeply rose pigmented form has been obtained from hedgehog quills.

Perfect States - There are two species of Arthroderma included under T. terrestre. Both are heterothallic. A. quadrifidum may be the more common species and includes the red hedgehog variant. The cells in the peridial hyphae in A. quadrifidum are asymmetric (dumbbell-shaped with lateral tubercles). The second species is A. lenticularum isolated to date from soil in California and India and is characterized by a yellower surface and subsurface of the thallus, slightly more beaded form of macroaleuriospores, and symmetrical (rather than asymmetrical) dumbbell-shaped cells in the peridial hyphae. A T. terrestre-like conidial state appears to characterize an undetermined number of other Arthroderma species as determined by mating experiments. These include

Trichophyton terrestre - Cont.

both heterothallic and homothallic forms. As many as four or five heterothallic species have been observed, but not characterized or named. Evidentally, care must be exercised in identifying fungi with the T. terrestre type of morphology, and mating experiments used if an exact specific identification is needed.

Critical Characteristics - (1) Micro- and macroaleuriospores, (2) Thallus characteristics, (3) Ascospores with either A. quadrifidum or A. lenticularum, (4) Form of the peridial hyphae seems to distinguish A. quadrifidum from A. lenticularum.

References:

Durie, E. B. and Frey, D., 1957. A New Species of Trichophyton from New South Wales, Mycologia, 49:401-411.

Marples, M. J. and Smith, J. M. B., 1962. Trichophyton terrestre as a Resident in Hedgehog Skin, Sabouraudia, 2:100-107.

Dawson, C. O. and Gentles, J. C., 1961. The Perfect States of Keratinomyces ajelloi Vanbreuseghem, Trichophyton terrestre Durie and Frey and Microsporum nanum Fuentes, Sabouraudia, 1:49-57.

Pore, R. S., Tsao, G. C., and Plunkett, O. A., 1965. A New Species of Arthroderma Established According to Biological Species Concepts, Mycologia, 57:969-973.

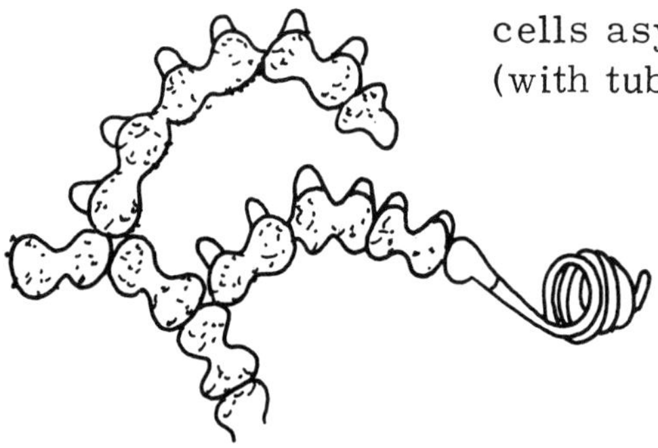

peridial hyphae of A. lenticularum

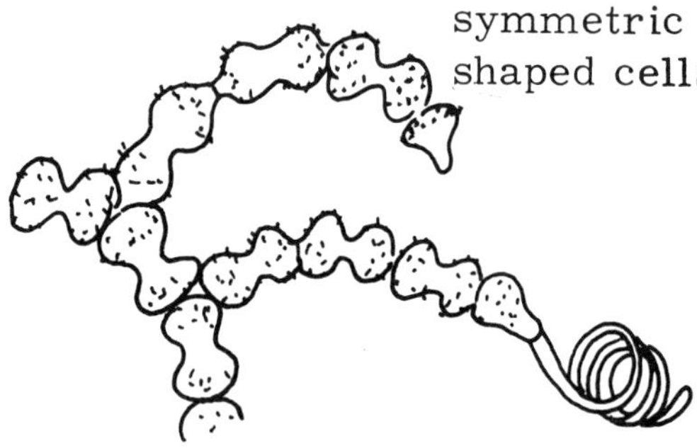

peridial hyphae of A. lenticularum

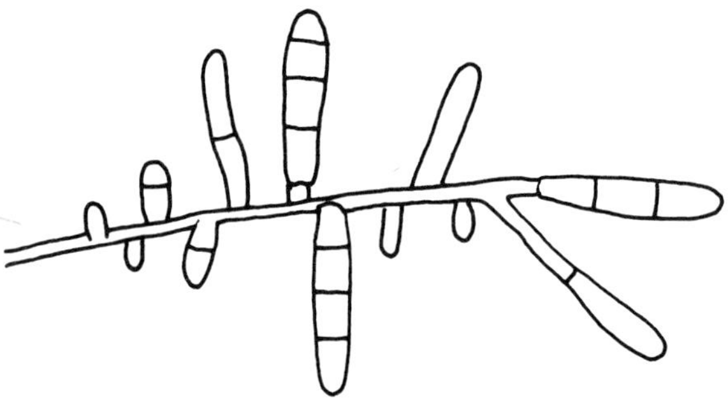

micro- and macroaleuriospores of A. lenticularum

Differences between the peridial hyphae of Arthroderma species (symmetric vs. asymmetric cells, etc.) may not be completely dependable.

Identification of Trichophyton georgii (Arthroderma ciferri)

Invasion of Hair - Not reported.

Clinical Disease - Not known to cause infections in man or lesions in animals.

Epidemiology - Probably geophilic.

Geographical Distribution - World-wide. Isolated from soil, mammalian pelage, feathers, and burrow nests of bank dwelling birds.

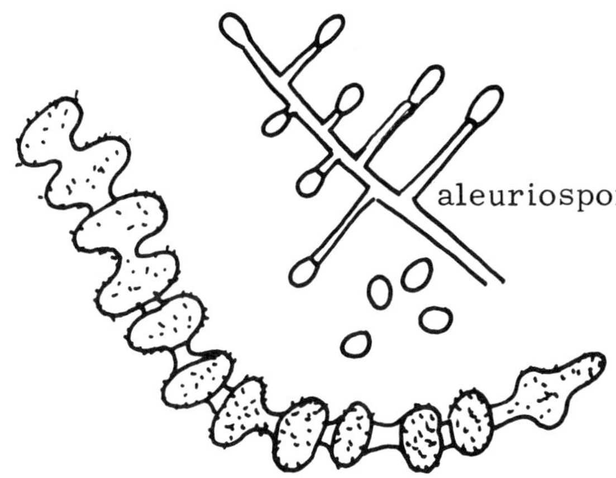

Appearance of Thallus - Thallus flat, with a carpet-like fluffy to powdery surface, red brown to lilac brown, resembling somewhat (but paler than) the red pigmented type of Arthroderma quadrifidum. Underside of thallus brown marked with brick red. Plate IV.

Microscopic Morphology - Clavate microaleuriospores resemble those of T. terrestre but smaller and rounder, size 2.0 - 2.4μ X 4.2 - 6.4μ as compared to 3.5 X 7 in T. terrestre. Some microaleuriospores may have one or two septa, but lateral macroaleuriospores of the T. terrestre type are not formed (see T. terrestre and T. thuringiense).* This homothallic species produces cleistothecia spontaneously on soil-hair substrate. The cells of the peridial hyphae are symmetrical dumbbell shaped as in A. uncinatum.

Special Nutritional Requirements - None reported.

Variants - Varsavsky and Ajello examined 11 red-pigmented T. terrestre-like fungi from soil and animal hair and found two isolates of T. ciferii, one of A. quadrifidum (new Zealand), one of an undescribed heterothallic Arthroderma sp. (Georgia, USA), and six additional isolates from Czechoslovakia and USA which were indeterminate since they formed unfertile cleistothecia. See also Chrysosporium with which this species shares the property of not producing macroaleuriospores.

Perfect State - Arthroderma ciferri (homothallic) (see microscopic morphology).

Special Media - Not required.

Critical Characteristics - (1) Microscopic morphology, (2) Morphology of thallus, (3) Homothallic, fertile cleistothecia from single ascospore, (4) Peridial hypha.

References:

Varsavsky, E. and Ajello, L., 1964. The Perfect and Imperfect Forms of a New Keratinophilic Fungus Arthroderma ciferri sp. nov; Trichophyton georgii sp. nov., Rivista di Pathologia Vegetale 4:351-364.

* The absence of macroaleuriospores might be argued to fit Chrysosporium.

Identification of Trichophyton gloriae

see also title page

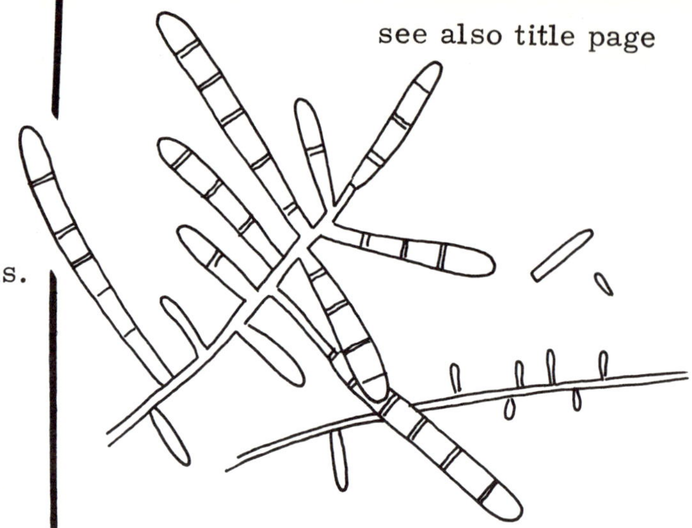

macro- and microaleuriospores

Invasion of Hair - Not described.

Clinical Disease - Not known to cause infections in man or lesions in animals.

Epidemiology - Isolated from soil in North America.

Geographical Distribution - To date, isolated from arid regions in California, Arizona, New Mexico, USA (lower Sonoran life zone) and also from soil in Canada.

Appearance of Thallus - A flat, downy to powdery thallus, varying from white, cream or yellowish to a distinctive cinnamon (color of macroaleuriospores in mass) suggestive of T. ajelloi. Radial grooves may be present. Undersurface of thallus becoming chrome yellow. Plate IV.

Microscopic Morphology - Macroaleuriospores narrow, varying in size and shape from one celled, slightly spindle shaped or rod like, to long cylindrical with up to 10 cells, resembling those of T. rubrum. Macroaleuriospores are usually abundant, occuring mainly on the terminal hyphal branches where they are arranged laterally in groups and clusters of varying size. In slide cultures, clusters of up to 40 macroaleuriospores may assume a spoke-like appearance. In mounts from agar plates the appearance is suggestive of T. terrestre. Rather small pyriform microaleuriospores are also present laterally on the hyphae and are frequently clearly differentiated from the small linear one-celled macroaleuriospore elements. In some cultures these small microaleuriospores may be the predominant microscopic feature. In others the macroaleuriospores appear to be replaced by chains of arthroaleuriospores suggestive of the morphology of Coccidioides immitis or the fungus genus Malbranchea.

Special Nutritional Requirements - None reported.

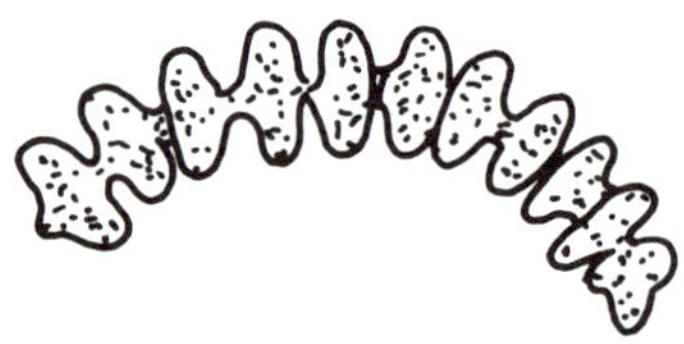

Variants - None reported.

peridial hypha of A. gloriae

Perfect State - Arthroderma gloriae (heterothallic), cells of peridial hyphae mainly symmetrical dumbbell shaped.

arthroaleuriospores

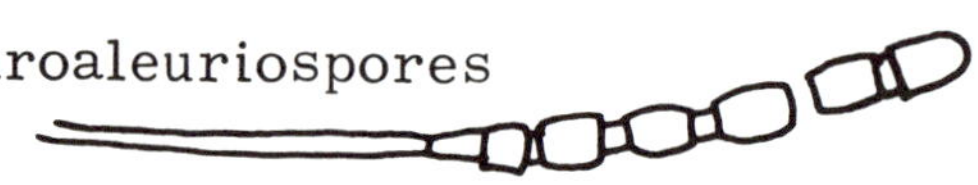

Special Media - Not required.

Critical Characteristics - (1) Macro- and microaleuriospores, (2) Appearance of thallus, (3) Ascospores with tester strains of A. gloriae, an important confirmation in view of the variable morphology.

References:

Ajello, L. and Cheng, S.Y., 1967. A New Geophilic Trichophyton, Mycologia 59:255-263

Identification of Trichophyton vanbreuseghemii

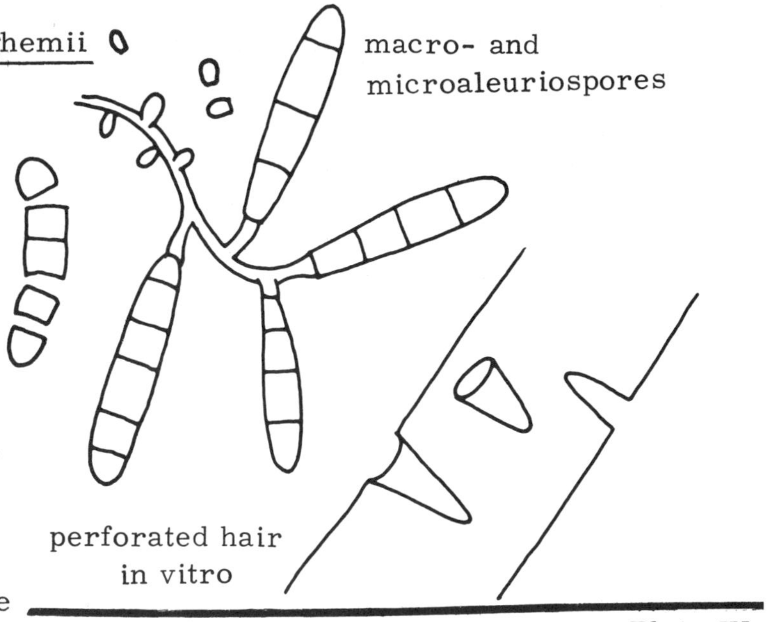

Invasion of Hair - Ectothrix in guinea pig. Perforates hair in vitro.

Clinical Disease - Dermatophytosis on hand of a forestry worker.

Epidemiology - Present in soil.

Geographical Distribution - Probably world-wide. Reports from North Africa, Europe, and Canada.

Appearance of Thallus - A warm buff colored thallus with the texture of fine glove leather, usually with central folds. A more powdery form is also seen. Plate IV.

Microscopic Morphology - The macroaleuriospores are characteristically plump, thin-walled, and cylindrical or club-shaped with rounded ends, and are produced in small clusters suggestive of T. ajelloi. The cells of the macroaleuriospores tend to separate when mature. Microaleuriospores are club-shaped, stubby with broad attachment scars, and produced mainly along the hyphae.

Special Nutritional Requirements - None.

Variants - Occurs naturally in powdery or velvety-fluffy types which segregate as genetic alleles.

Perfect State - Arthroderma gertleri (heterothallic).

Special Media - Not required.

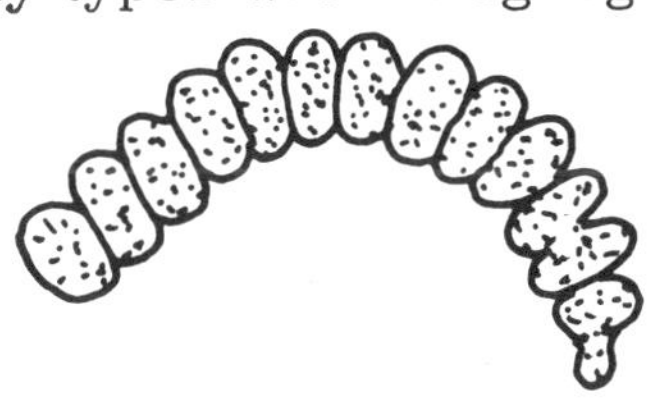
peridial hypha
of A. gertleri

Critical Characteristics - (1) Microscopic morphology, (2) Buff color of thallus, (3) Ascospores with tester strains of A. gertleri.

References:

Rioux, J. A., Jarry, D. T., and Juminer, B., 1964. Un Nouveau Dermatophyte Isolé du Sol: Trichophyton vanbreuseghemii n. sp., Naturalia Monspeliensia, Ser. Botznique, 16:153-162.

Rioux, J. A., Jarry, D. T., Jarry, D. M., and Juminer, B., 1966. Trichophyton vanbreuseghemii Rioux, Jarry et Juminer, 1964 Observations complémentaires, Ann. de Parasitologie (Paris), 41:195-201.

Böhme, H., 1967. Arthroderma gertleri sp. nov., die perfekte Form von Trichophyton vanbreuseghemii Rioux, Jarry et Juminer, Mykosen 10: 247-252.

Böhme, H. and Hejtmankova-Uhrova, N., 1968. Habituelle Unterschiede und Sexuelle Kompatibilität bei Arthroderma gertleri Böhme, Mykosen 11: 573-578.

Identification of Trichophyton simii

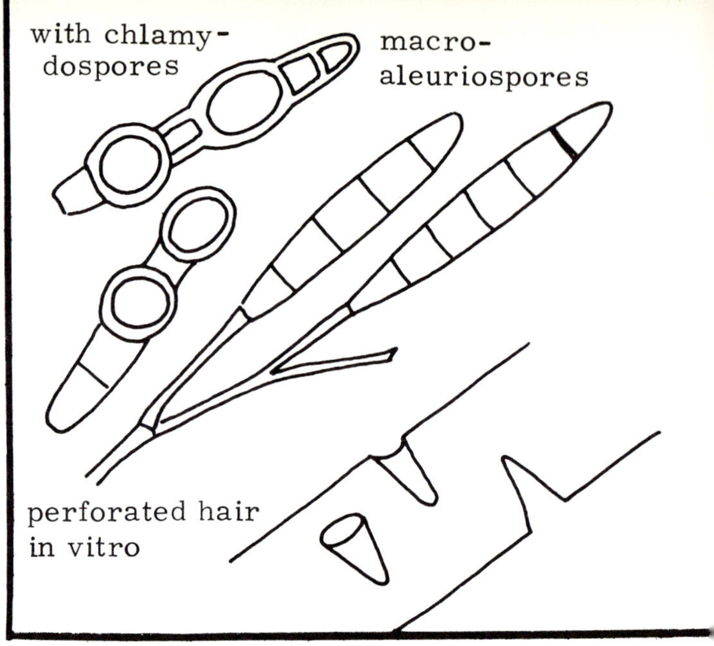

Invasion of Hair - In guinea pigs parasitism of hair occurs with large endothrix as well as ectothrix spores in chains. There is a bright green fluorescence of the parasitized hair. Parasitism of hair in man has not been reported and in monkeys it is minimal, but with some green fluorescence. The fungus perforates hair in vitro.

Clinical Disease - Occasional to frequent tinea corporis in man which may or may not be somewhat inflammatory and persistent, and apparently contracted rather easily from infected animals. Hair not involved. In monkey, silvery scaling lesions with minimal hair involvement (in contrast to T. mentagrophytes). In poultry, white papulomatous plaques, affecting the comb and wattles, similar to infections with T. (M?) gallinae, but possibly producing more inflammatory involvement of the corneum and local necrosis.

Epidemiology - Infects rhesus monkeys and chickens commonly, and also isolated from soil and various small mammals in India. Apparently a zoophilic or geophilic species.

Geographical Distribution - Restricted to India, but also reported from an African chimpanzee in a Tokyo Zoo. Although commonly associated with primates and chickens, the fungus may have a small mammal host (as yet undiscovered).

Appearance of Thallus - A rapidly growing flat or slightly folded and raised thallus. Densely to heavily powdery suggestive of T. mentagrophytes or M. audouinii var. langeronii. Surface white to yellow-buff or pink (sometimes splotched with these colors), with a madder-rose, yellowish, or vinaceous (reddish-brown) color developing beneath the thallus. May develop both powdery and wart-like masses composed of macroaleuriospores. Plate IV.

Microscopic Morphology - Typically produces large numbers of smooth-walled well formed club-shaped or elongate macroaleuriospores in loose clusters. Macroaleuriospores develop enlarged chlamydospore-like cells and also break into segments at maturity. In young macroaleuriospores this is manifested by the septa which are frequently unevenly spaced, creating large cells and small cells which may stain unequally with cotton blue. Narrow, elongate, pyriform to peg-shaped microaleuriospores are also present, arranged along the hyphae and on terminal branches but not in conspicuous clusters. In young thalli the microscopic appearance is, therefore, the reverse of that usually obtained with T. mentagrophytes with respect to the relative numbers and arrangement

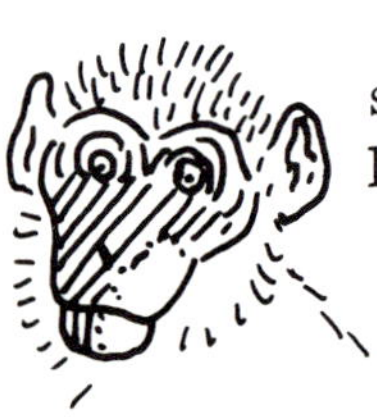

silvery scaling
lesion on Macaca

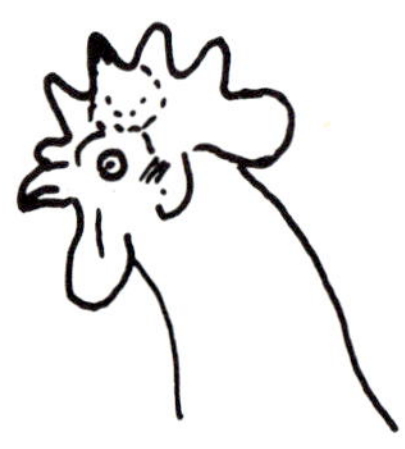

necrotic lesion
on chicken comb

Trichophyton simii - Cont.

of macro- and microaleuriospores. The individual macroaleuriospores may resemble those of T. mentagrophytes which under adverse conditions in culture may also develop internal chlamydospores and beaded forms. As in T. mentagrophytes spirals may be present. In some mature cultures more abundant pyriform microaleuriospores and elongate disarticulated macroaleuriospores may be suggestive of T. rubrum.

Special Nutritional Requirements - None reported.

Variants - Not reported.

Perfect State - Arthroderma simii (heterothallic), rather easily produced on soil with horse hair or feathers. A simii tester strains can be used to determine the mating type of other dermatophytes. See illustration page 43.

Special Media - Not required.

Critical Characteristics - (1) Macroaleuriospores, (2) Production of severe fluorescent ringworm in guinea pigs, (3) Thallus characteristics, (4) Ascospores with tester strain of Arthroderma simii, (5) To date all isolations traced geographically to India or to primates of Indian or African origin.

References:

Stockdale, P.M., Mackenzie, D.W.R., and Austwick, P.K.C., 1965. Arthroderma simii sp. nov., The Perfect State of Trichophyton simii (Pinoy) comb. nov., Sabouraudia 4:112-123.

Rippon, J.W., Eng, A., and Malkinson, F.D., 1968. Trichophyton simii Infection in the United States, Arch. Derm. 98:615-619.

Gugnani, H.C., Mulay, D.N., and Murty, D.K., 1967. Fungus Flora of Dermatophytosis and Trichophyton simii Infections in Northern India, Indian J. Derm. and Venerol. 33:73-82.

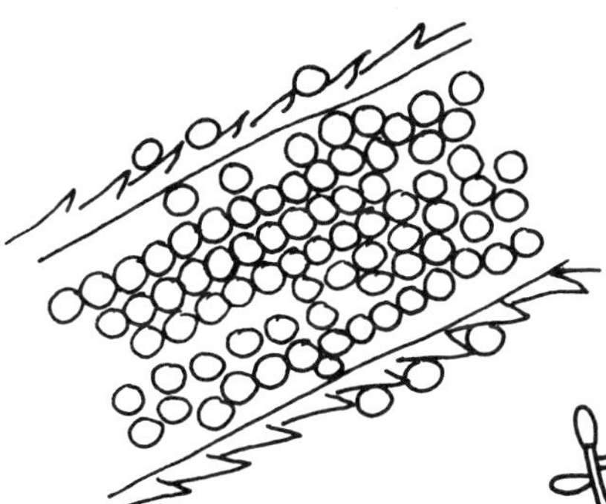

parasitized guinea pig hair

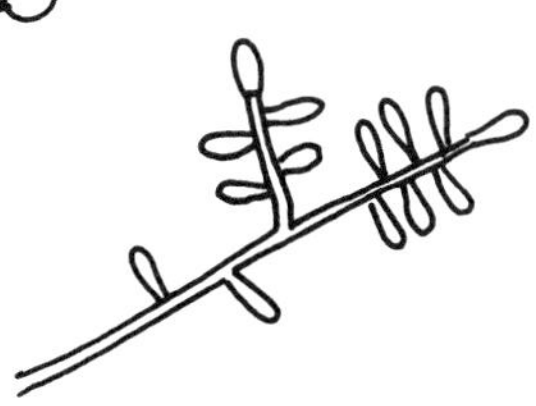

microaleuriospores

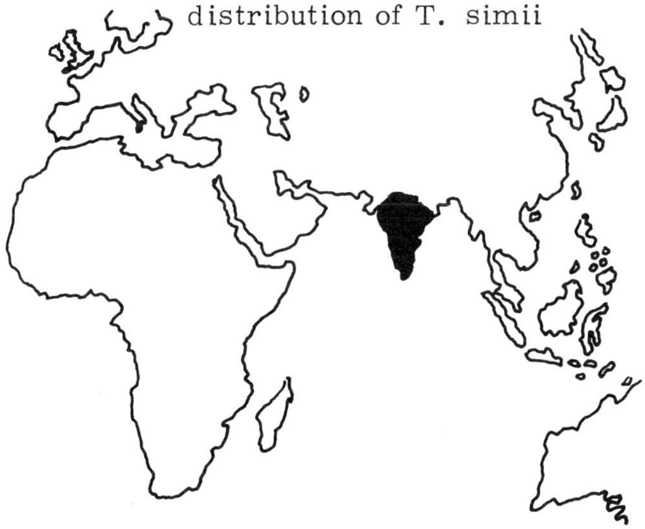

distribution of T. simii

Identification of Trichophyton mentagrophytes.

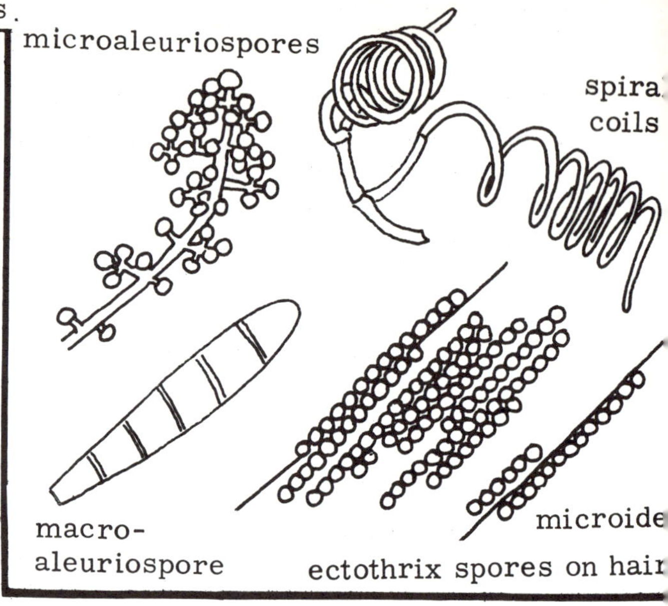

Invasion of Hair - Zoophilic types produce ectothrix chains of moderate size spores on the surface of the hair. The spores are visible under the low power objective of the microscope. Hair not fluorescent. The zoophilic type var. quinkeanum has less tendency to invade hair and in the guinea pig may produce endothrix invasion with fluorescence suggestive of T. simii. The homophilic interdigitale variety usually does not invade hair. All varieties of T. mentagrophytes perforate hair in vitro.

Clinical Disease - Tinea capitis, tinea corporis, tinea barbae, tinea cruris, tinea pedis and onychomycosis, including direct infection of the nail plate (white spot nail disease). Isolated lesions of the scalp, beard and on the body surface are usually highly inflammatory and often undergo rapid resolution. May simulate furunculosis. T. mentagrophytes is still the commonest cause of tinea pedis, which is chronic and resembles that caused by other species. However, it is a rare cause of tinea cruris, the commonest cause being T. rubrum. Zoophilic strains may produce isolated inflammatory lesions frequently with deep involvement of the hair follicles or a widespread tinea corporis suggestive of T. rubrum and E. floccosum. One form (var. quinckeanum) is associated with favus-like scutula in mice and occasionally in man. May be associated with veterinary syndrome "Collie Nose" (J. C. Blakemore, D.V.M.).

Epidemiology - Infections are widespread among animals. The usual cause of epizootics of ringworm in laboratory animals and ringworm in horses in the USA. The zoophilic form of T. mentagrophytes is highly infectious and capable of transfer to man, usually producing solitary inflammatory lesions. Infections may occur in persons handling laboratory cultures and infected laboratory animals.

An anthropophilic type of T. mentagrophytes is associated with tinea pedis and less frequently tinea cruris in man. This type is difficult to inoculate into laboratory animals and produces a milder lesion without invasion of the hair. The anthropophilic form can be transformed into the zoophilic form by serial transfer on the skin of guinea pigs.

Geographical Distribution - World-wide. A powdery, zoophilic type is present in South East Asia which produces widespread multiple infections, frequently with deep follicular involvement, particularly in American and British military personnel.

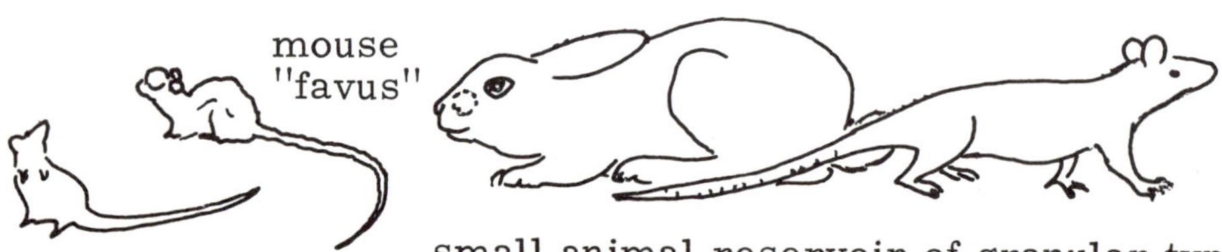

small animal reservoir of granular type

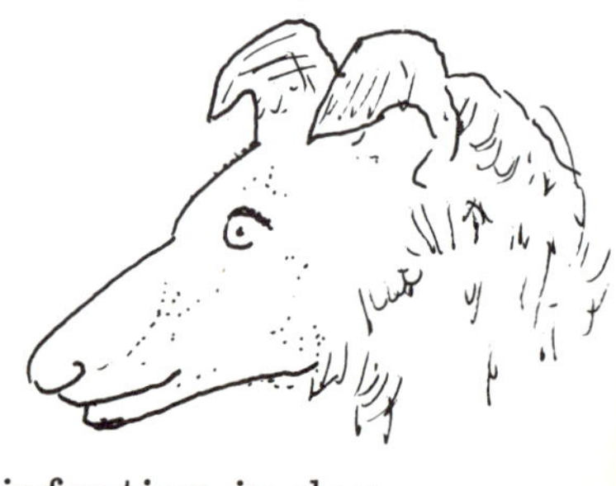

infection in dog

Trichophyton mentagrophytes - Cont.

Appearance of Thallus - The zoophilic form characteristically produces a flat thallus with a cream or yellowish buff powdery surface. The powder which has the appearance of face powder sprinkled in concentric rings and rays consists mainly of large clusters of microaleuriospores. Some strains develop dark red pigment on the underside of the thallus rather than the more usual brown-tan color. Others are bright yellow beneath.

The tinea pedis or anthropophilic form usually grows out on Sabouraud's agar as a flat, densely downy thallus with a tint of cream colored spores. Older colonies may become pink-tinted. Close observation of the thallus will usually reveal more or less of a powdery substrate which can be confirmed by microscopic demonstration of clustered microaleuriospores. Transferred to potato dextrose agar a characteristic stellate powdery thallus is produced. Strains of the tinea pedis type actually exhibit a wide range of variation in the degree to which they approach the typical powdery appearance of zoophilic isolates. All thalli of T. mentagrophytes rapidly become pleomorphic developing a dense fluff with little or no sporulation. Plates II and IV.

Microscopic Morphology - The zoophilic form is very rich in numbers and types of microscopic structures, the downy anthropophilic form less so, and pleomorphic strains essentially sterile. Small spherical microaleuriospores produced in clusters resembling unripe grapes are characteristic of T. mentagrophytes. In downy strains the clusters are reduced in size and number and tear-shaped microaleuriospores may be seen which are more difficult to distinguish from those of T. rubrum.

Macroaleuriospores may be present in some numbers particularly in zoophilic strains. These are usually well-formed and club-shaped, present in association with the microaleuriospores and other structures, usually rather early in the life of the thallus. The cigar shape and narrow attachments to the vegetative hyphae will serve to distinguish the macroaleuriospores from those of T. rubrum. Many strains also produce an abundance of coiled spirals. Although these are not unique to T. mentagrophytes they are not often present in such abundance in other dermatophyte cultures.

The microaleuriospores, macroaleuriospores, and spirals in the granular strains are often associated with antler-like structures resembling the peridial hyphae of the perfect form.

Special Nutritional Requirements - None reported.

Variants - The many variations in the powdery surface, degree of folding of the thallus, and pigment formation of T. mentagrophytes resulted in many synonyms now obsolete. A glabrous to white fluffy thallus with a deep yellow to orange pigment on the underside is occasionally isolated from tinea pedis. Many nodular bodies and relatively few microaleuriospores are seen on microscopic examination. These isolates have been named variety nodulare. Mutagenic agents induce variants which may superficially resemble T. violaceum and other species. The var. quinckeanum form associated with mouse favus may have a plicated, sometimes pigmented thallus, and has lateral tear-shaped microaleuriospores only. Yellow granular forms occur in Africa which suggest T. erinacei.

Trichophyton mentagrophytes - Cont.

Perfect State - Arthroderma benhamiae, heterothallic. All major types, viz. zoophilic granular strains (var. granulosum), var. inderdigitale (the anthropophilic tinea pedis form), var. quinkeanum, and var. nodulare, mate with tester strains of Arthroderma benhamiae. Some granular isolates from small mammals and soil do not mate with A. benhamiae and suggest the existence of other species. T. erinacei has been separated from T. mentagrophytes on this basis.

Special Media - Potato dextrose agar is useful in separating the tinea pedis type of T. mentagrophytes from T. rubrum. Most strains of the latter species develop a deep rose-red pigment on this medium which contrasts markedly with stellate powdery thallus of T. mentagrophytes. The pigment of red strains of T. mentagrophytes is not produced on corn meal agar. When grown on autoclaved hair, mentagrophytes perforates the hair. T. rubrum does not. T. mentagrophytes also has greater urease activity than most isolates of T. rubrum.

Critical Characteristics - (1) Small round microaleuriospores in clusters, (2) Spirals in the presence of typical microaleuriospores, (3) Well formed macroaleuriospores, (4) Morphology of thallus, (5) Ability to perforate hairs in vitro, (6) Ascospores with tester strains of A. benhamiae.

References:

Georg, L.K., 1954. The Relationship Between the Downy and Granular Forms of Trichophyton mentagrophytes, J. Invest. Derm., 23:123-141.

LaTouche, C.J., 1960. Mouse Favus Due to Trichophyton quinckeanum (Zopf) Macleod and Muende, A Reappraisal in the Light of Recent Investigations. IV. Mycopathologica, 13:33-47.

Ajello, L. and Cheng, S., 1967. The Perfect State of Trichophyton mentagrophytes, Sabouraudia, 5:230-234.

Donald, G.F. and Brown, G. (with assistance of Chappell, W.T.), 1964. T. mentagrophytes and T. mentagrophytes var. quinkeanum Infections of South Australian Mice, Aust. J. Derm., 7:133.

Padhye, A. A. and Carmichael, J.W., 1969. Mating Behaviour of Trichophyton mentagrophytes Varieties Paired with Arthroderma benhamiae Mating Types, Sabouraudia, 7:178-181.

Marais, V. and Olivier, D.L., 1965. Isolation of Trichophyton mentagrophytes from a Porcupine, Sabouraudia, 4·49-52.

Georg, L.K. and Maechling, E.H., 1949. Trichophyton mentagrophytes (variety nodular), J. Invest. Derm., 13:339-350.

Blank, H., Taplin, D., and Zaias, N., 1969. Cutaneous Trichophyton mentagrophytes Infections in Vietnam, Arch. Derm. 99:135-144.

Trichophyton mentagrophytes - Cont.

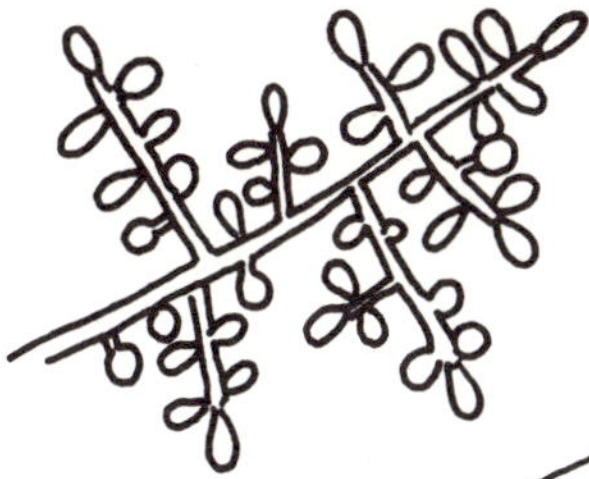

atypical clusters with mostly clavate microaleuriospores

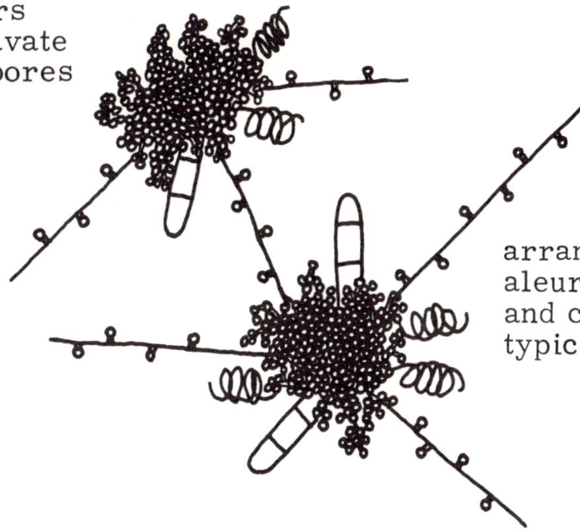

arrangement of aleuriospores and coils in a typical thallus

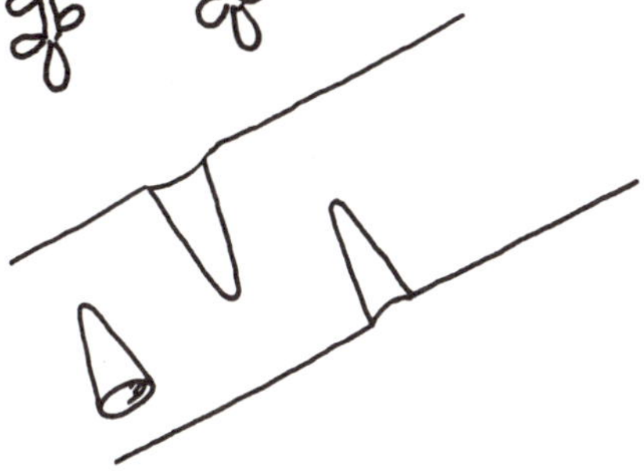

perforated hair in vitro

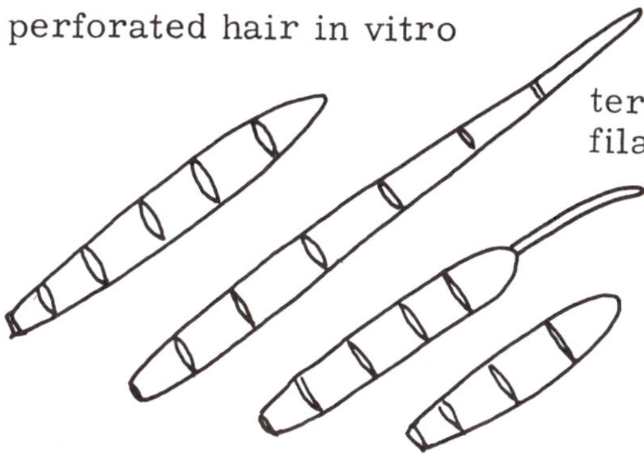

macroaleuriospores

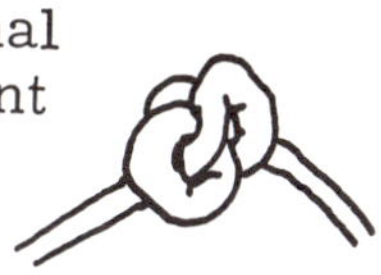

nodular organ

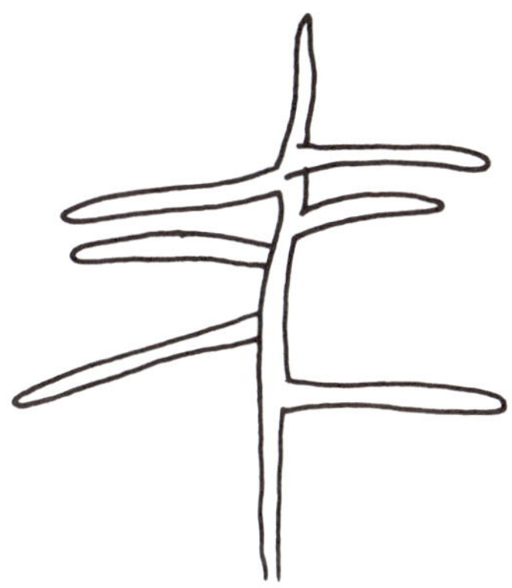

antler-like hyphae

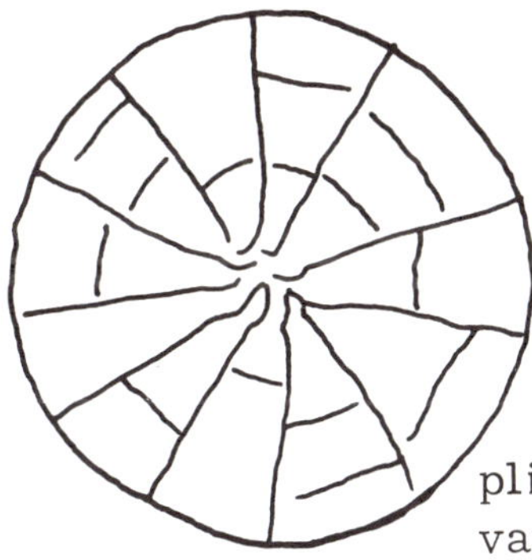

plicated thallus of var. quinkeanum

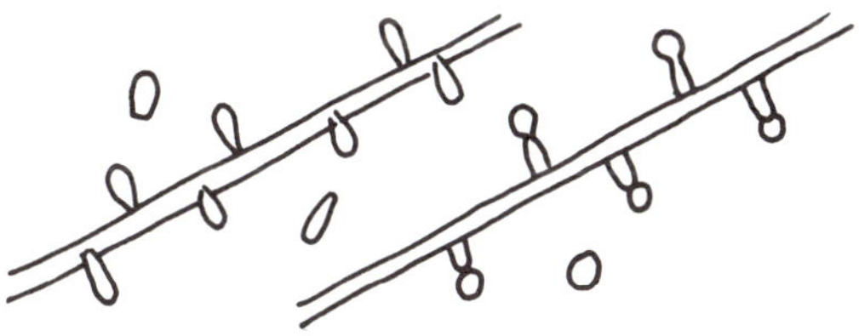

lateral microaleuriospores

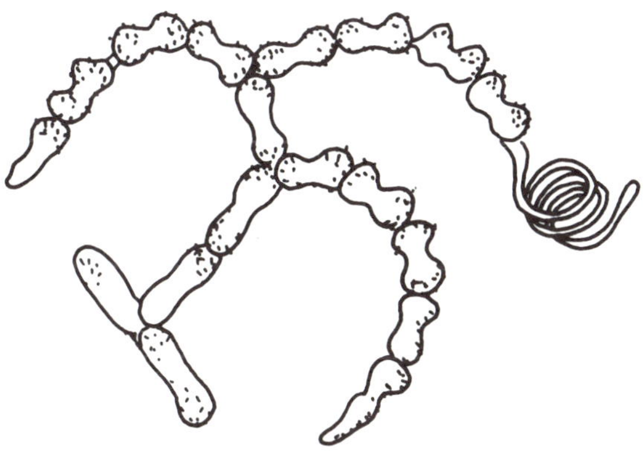

peridial hyphae of A. benhamiae

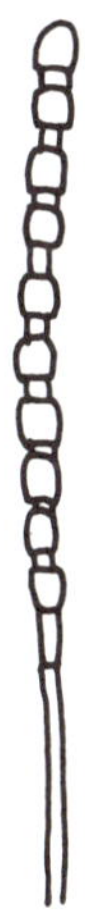

arthroaleuriospores

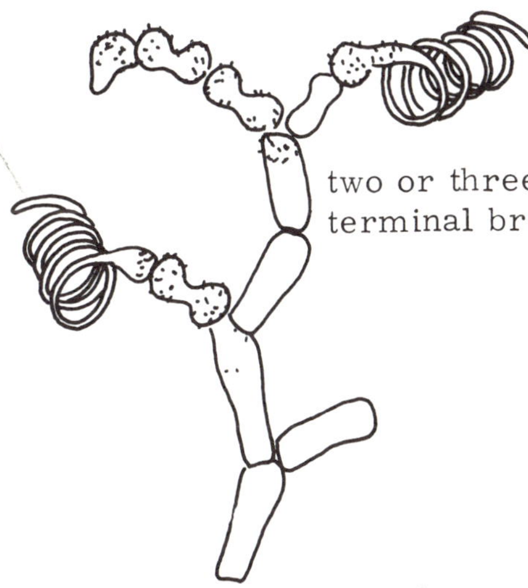

peridial hyphae of A. simii (see page 38)

Identification of Trichophyton erinacei

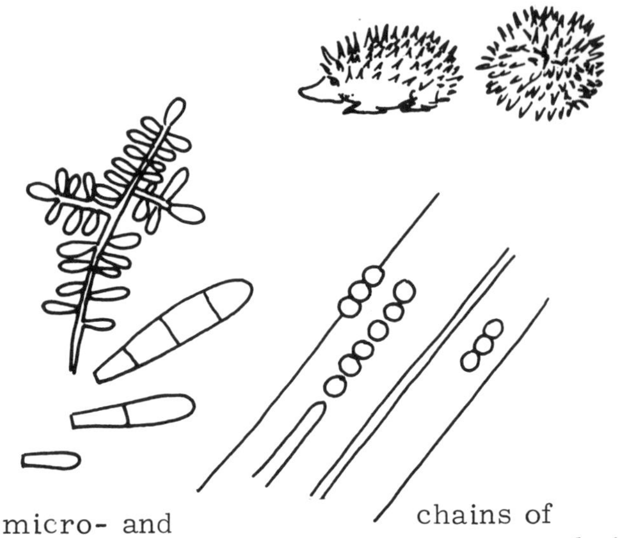

Invasion of Hair - Ectothrix. In guinea pig infections arthrospores may be inside the hair as well as outside.

Clinical Disease - Isolated lesions which tend to be eczematous and most frequently on lower limbs and on hands and wrists. Can cause tinea capitis, tinea barbae, and toe and fingernail infections.

Epidemiology - This species and the red form of T. terrestre are characteristically associated with the hedgehog. In contrast to T. terrestre which is present saprophytically on the hedgehog quills, T. erinacei may produce lesions about the nose and other parts of the hedgehog, sometimes associated with epidermal mites. T. erinacei has in fact been isolated from mites and their excreta and could be transmitted by mites. Prevalence of infections in wild hedgehogs may approach 50 percent of animals.

Geographical Distribution - Distribution confined to and presumably coextensive with that of hedgehogs. To date T. erinacei has been isolated from New Zealand, the British Isles, and continental Europe.

Appearance of Thallus - A flat, white to ivory white, lightly powdery thallus with a clear yellow diffusing pigment beneath. Plate II.

Microscopic Morphology - Microaleuriospores are club-shaped rather than spherical, and produced abundantly on terminal hyphal branches. Macroaleuriospores are club-shaped, similar to T. mentagrophytes, but shorter with fewer cells and with forms intermediate in appearance between microaleuriospores and macroaleuriospores. Spirals may be present in old cultures.

Special Nutritional Requirements - Not reported.

Variants - None reported.

Perfect State - Unknown. Does not mate with A. benhamiae mating types. To date all strains tested against A. simii have been (+) mating type.

Special Media - T. erinacei may be distinguished from T. mentagrophytes by its inability to grow at pH 4, and lack of urease (see methods).

Critical Characteristics - (1) White powdery thallus, yellow beneath, (2) Microscopic morphology, (3) Failure to grow at pH 4 and hydrolyze urea, (4) Failure to produce ascospores with tester strains of A. benhamiae.

References:

Smith, J.M.B. and Marples, M.J., 1963. Trichophyton mentagrophytes var. erinacei, Sabouraudia, 3:1-10.

Identification of Trichophyton equinum

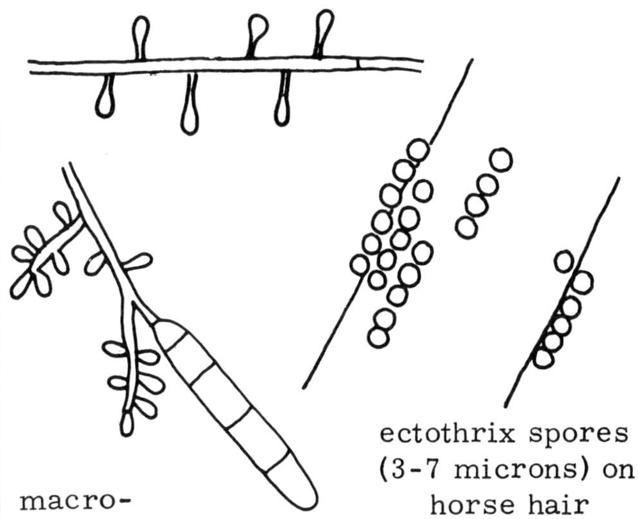

Invasion of Hair - In horse, relatively large ectothrix spores in chains.

Clinical Disease - Rare infections with both nicotinic acid requiring and autotrophic variants in man. In horses, papular, crusting, multiple lesions, involving skin and hair.

Epidemiology - A specific cause of ringworm in horses. Trichophyton mentagrophytes also commonly causes ringworm in horses resulting in some confusion of the two species.

Geographical Distribution - World-wide (recent report from Africa). In Australia and New Zealand strains isolated to date do not require nicotinic acid.

Appearance of Thallus - Thallus rather similar to a fluffy type of T. mentagrophytes, usually with a clear, deep yellow pigment on the underside which may be visible from above as a yellow perimeter. The center of the thallus is frequently reddish and may become deep orange brown to dark brown as the thallus ages. May produce brown diffusing pigment. The edge of the thallus is often noticeably ragged compared to T. mentagrophytes and the surface tends to become brownish or pink and cracked with age. Plate II.

Microscopic Morphology - Typically pyriform to spherical stalked microaleuriospores along the hyphae. Less frequently the microaleuriospores are clustered with clavate macroaleuriospores of the Trichophyton type, similar to T. mentagrophytes and T. erinacei. Nodular organs which often characterize the yellow pigmented nodular variety of T. mentagrophytes are not abundant.

Special Nutritional Requirements - Except for the New Zealand and Australian strains the fungus requires nicotinic acid (niacin) in the medium. It also has been reported to grow selectively on horse hair in vitro and will not grow on human hair in vitro. This has not proven to be due to its niacin requirement and may not be a reliable differential characteristic.

Variants - T. equinum var. autotrophicum (otherwise typical) does not require nicotinic acid.

Perfect State - Not reported.

Special Media - Demonstration of requirement when it exists for niacin is specific and diagnostic.

Trichophyton equinum - Cont.

Critical Characteristics - (1) Characteristics of thallus, (2) Microscopic appearance, (3) Niacin requirement, and (4) Pathogenicity for the horse.

References:

Georg, L.K., Kaplan, W., and Camp, L.B., 1957. Trichophyton equinum - A Re-evaluation of its Taxonomic Status, J. Invest. Dermat., 29:27-37.

Smith, J.M.B., Jolly, R.D., Georg, L.K., and Connole, M.D., 1968. Trichophyton equinum var. autotrophicum; Its Characteristics and Geographical Distribution, Sabouraudia 6:296-304.

TRICHOPHYTON SPECIES COMMON IN VETERINARY MEDICINE

T. mentagrophytes (small animals and farm animals) readily transmitted to man.

T. equinum (horse) rarely transmitted to man.

T. verrucosum (cattle) frequently transmitted to man and other animals.

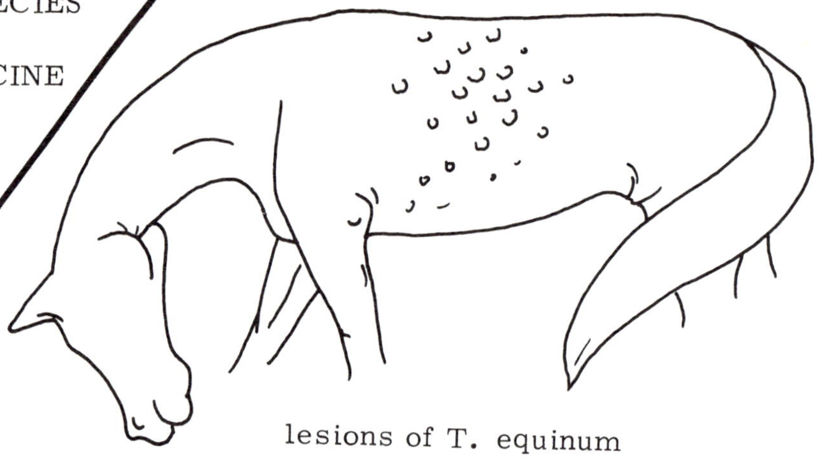

lesions of T. equinum

Test for Nicotinic Acid (Niacin) Requirement of Heterotrophic Isolates of T. equinum

A. Vitamin-Free Acid-Hydrolyzed Casein (2.5 mg)
(or 25 ml of a 10 percent solution of same)

glucose	40 grams
$MgSO_4$	0.1 grams
KH_2PO_4	1.8 grams
agar	20 grams
dist. water	1000 mls

Autoclave (120°C, 15 minutes)

B. Nicotinic Acid Solution

nicotinic acid	10.0 mgs
dist. water	100 mls

Autoclave (120°C, 10 minutes). Store at 5°C.

vit.-free cas. hydrol. medium	vit.-free cas. hydrol. medium with nicotinic acid
no growth of heterotrophic isolates of T. equinum	growth of all isolates of T. equinum

C. Add 2 ml of Solution B to 100 ml melted Basal Medium A and slant in tubes.
Inoculate slant of C and slant of control Basal Medium A with pinhead-size fragments of viable culture. Observe for growth. Re-check positive growth by one serial transfer to fresh test media.

Identification of Trichophyton verrucosum

Invasion of Hair - Markedly large ectothrix spores (5-10μ) in chains. Hair not fluorescent in man. Fluorescence of hair has been noted in cattle.

Clinical Disease - Highly inflammatory, isolated, scattered, or widespread ringworm lesions, usually involving the scalp, beard or exposed areas of the body. Frequently similar to zoophilic T. mentagrophytes.

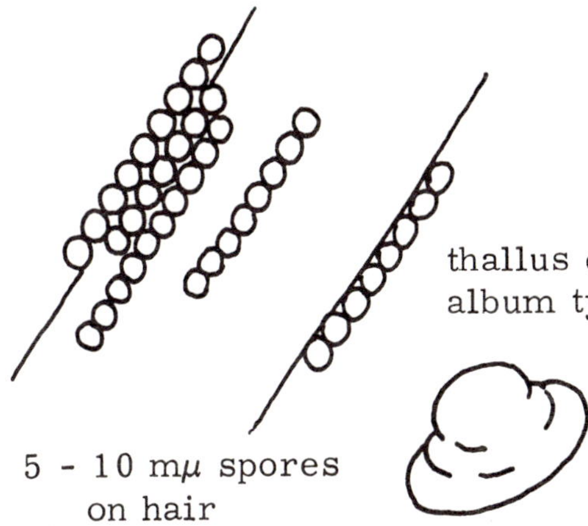

Epidemiology - The principle cause of ringworm in cattle. Infections in man usually contracted directly from cattle or infected fomites. In cattle, crusting lesions, particularly in late winter, and in calves, and in dairy breeds.

Geographical Distribution - World-wide.

Appearance of Thallus - Usually a white, very slow growing, glabrous thallus resembling T. schoenleinii, but heaped up and button-like rather than convoluted folding and spreading. Two additional variants occur; a flat, yellow, glabrous thallus (var. ochraceum) and a flat, slightly downy grey-white thallus (var discoides). On blood agar base enriched with thiamine and inositol (or yeast extract) thalli are more spreading, flat and slightly downy. Plate II .

Microscopic Morphology - On Sabouraud's agar tortuous hyphae are seen with antler-like branching suggesting T. schoenleinii but less often with the swollen 'nail head' tips. On blood agar base enriched with thiamine tear-shaped microaleuriospores are seen and less frequently macroaleuriospores which may have a rather characteristic rat tail or string bean shape.

Special Nutritional Requirements - All strains require thiamine. Many strains also require inositol. Unlike other dermatophytes growth is usually enhanced at 37°C.

Variants - The three principal variants 'album', 'ochraceum', and 'discoides' are described above. The typical forms are somewhat difficult to maintain in stock culture because of pleomorphic changes and tendency to sector. The fungus does not remain viable in the refrigerator.

Perfect State - Not reported. Structures resembling Arthroderma-type peridial hyphae have been reported.

Special Media - Absolute requirements for thiamine and usually inositol distinguish this species from T. schoenleinii and other glabrous dermatophytes. Aleuriospores may also be obtainable on enriched media.

Trichophyton verrucosum - Cont.

Critical Characteristics - (1) Morphology of thallus and requirement for thiamine and inositol, (2) Clinical lesion and history, (3) Megathrix sporulation on hair, (4) Grows slower than other common American dermatophytes, and (5) Improved growth at 37°C.

References:

Georg, L.K., 1950. The Relation of Nutrition to the Growth and Morphology of Trichophyton faviforme, Mycologia, 42:683.

var album

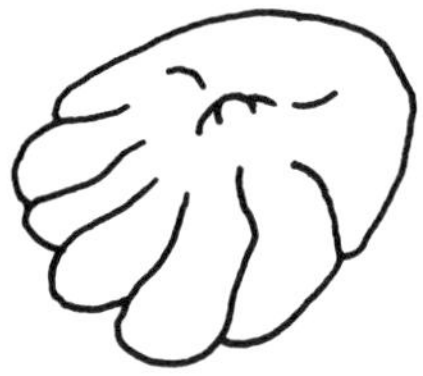

var ochraceum

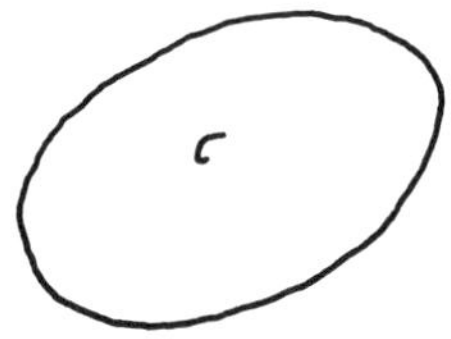

var discoides

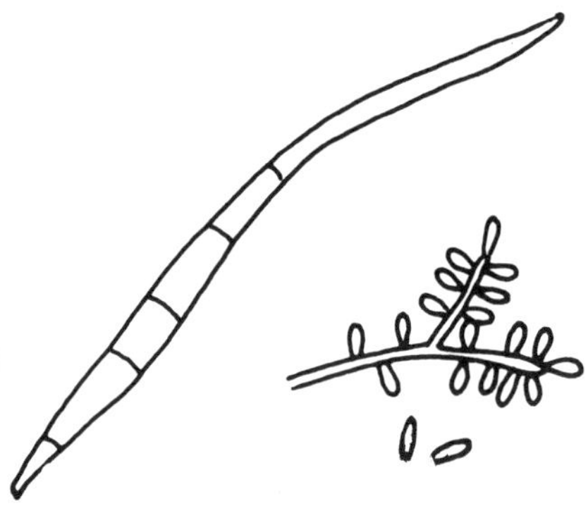

macro- and microaleuriospores produced in presence of thiamine and inosital

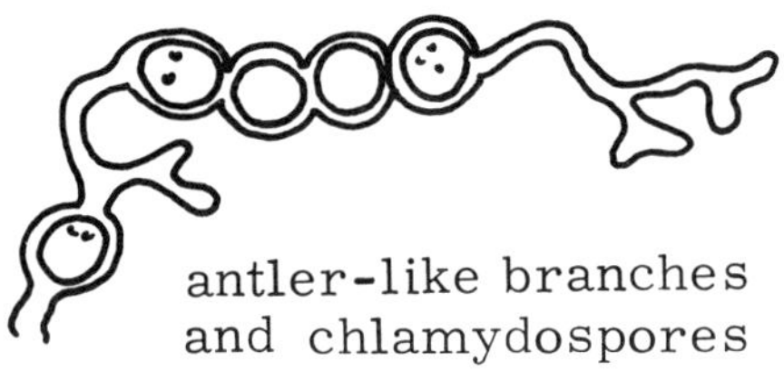

antler-like branches and chlamydospores

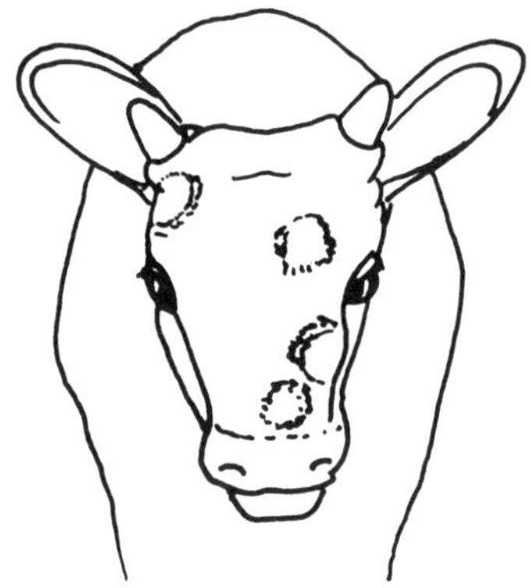

lesion of T. verrucosum

Test for Thiamine and Inositol Requirements of T. verrucosum

A. Basal Medium (Vitamin-Free Casein Hydrolysate Medium (see page 46).

B. Thiamine Solution

thiamine hydrochloride	10 mgs
distilled water (pH 4 - 5)	1000 mls

C. Inositol Solution

i-inositol	250 mgs
distilled water	100 mls

Sterilize vitamin solutions and procede and inoculate slants as on page 46.

vit.-free cas. hydrol. medium	vit.-free cas. hydrol. medium with thiamine	vit.-free cas. hydrol. medium with thiamine and inisotol
no growth	growth of some isolates	growth of all isolates

Identification of Trichophyton megninii

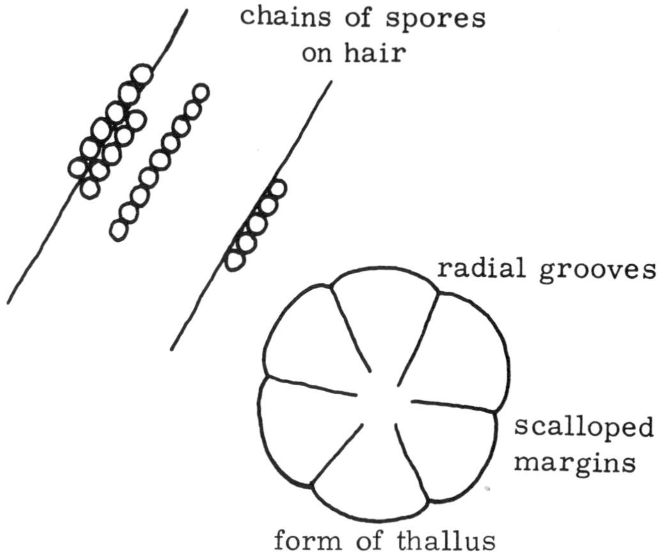

Invasion of Hair - Ectothrix, with moderate size spores in chains on surface of hair.

Clinical Disease - Primarily a cause of tinea barbae. Tinea corporis and tinea capitis less common.

Epidemiology - To date an anthropophilic species possibly spread by barber shops.

Geographical Distribution - This fungus is seen only in Europe and Africa (Burundi and North Africa). Particularly common in Portugal and Sardinia. It is not known in the Western Hemisphere.

Appearance of Thallus - Characteristically a fairly rapidly growing felt or suede-like colony with widely spaced radial grooves and a pink surface. Red pigment also develops under the thallus, but is not as intense as in most strains of T. rubrum and of a more claret than port-wine color. Plate II.

Microscopic Morphology - Pyriform to clavate microaleuriospores. Macroaleuriospores are infrequent and may be long and pencil shaped resembling those of T. rubrum. The microscopic features are not in themselves diagnostic.

Special Nutritional Requirements - T. megninii requires l-histidine for growth, otherwise suggestive of T. rubrum, T. gourvillii, and T. fluviomuniensis.

Variants - None described. Recent synonym, T. kuryangei.

Perfect State - Not known.

Special Media - May be distinguished from all other dermatophytes by its unique requirement for l-histidine.

Critical Characteristics - (1) Morphology of thallus, (2) Histidine requirement, (3) Rare, unknown, or misidentified outside Europe and Africa.

Test for Histidine Requirement

A. Substitute 1.5 gm NH_4NO_3 for casein hydrolysate, page 46.

B. Histidine Solution
l-histidine, 150 mg
dist. water, 100 ml

Follow procedure on page 46.

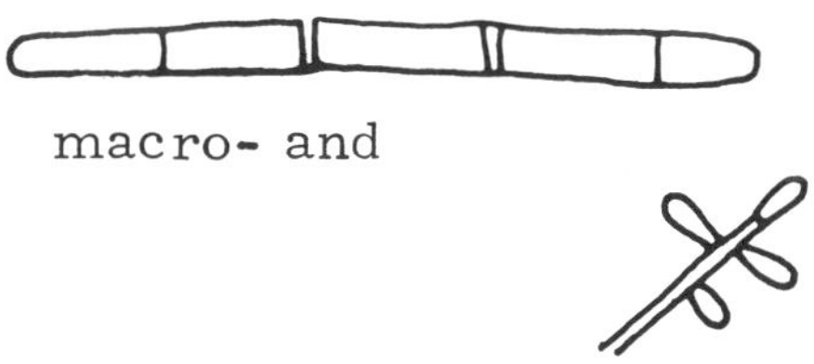

NH_4NO_3 medium	NH_4NO_3 medium with histidine
no growth	growth

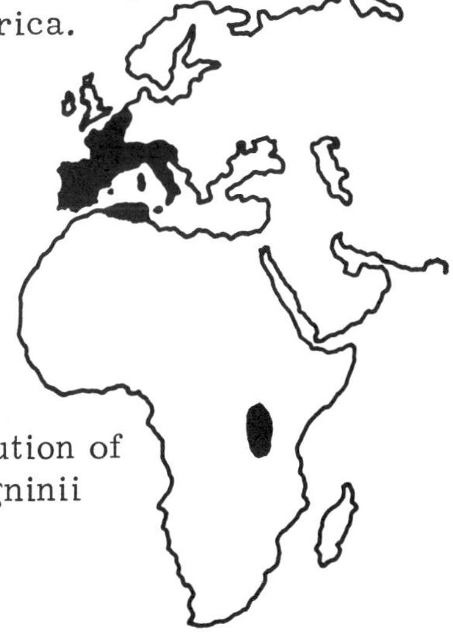

distribution of T. megninii

Identification of Trichophyton rubrum

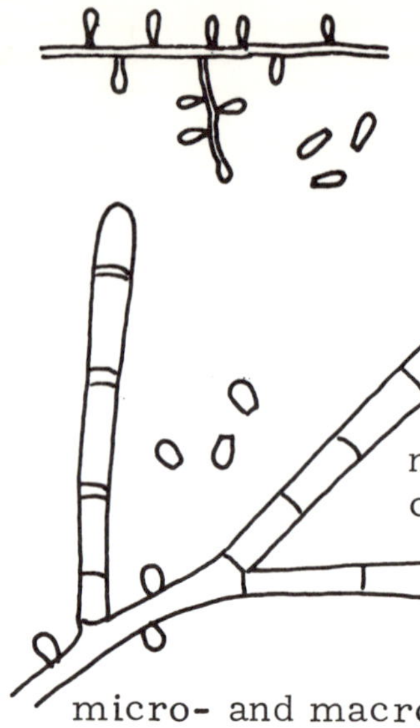

Invasion of Hair - Reported both as ectothrix chains of rather large spores and as typical endothrix. Not fluorescent. Scalp infections rare. Usually does not form perforating organs in vitro and does not invade the nail plate (see T. mentagrophytes).

Clinical Disease - Primarily a cause of tinea corporis, tinea pedis, tinea manum and onychomycosis. Tinea corporis lesions are notably chronic and spreading often with red indurated margin and wide central clearing. In rare cases may simulate tinea imbricata. Commonest cause of tinea manum. Tinea capitis rare but has been reported as typical endothrix T. tonsurans type, tinea barbae more frequent. Granulomatous, deep follicular lesions (Majocchi's granuloma) are sometimes seen, usually involving the legs of young women.

Epidemiology - A widespread anthropophilic species which appears to be increasing everywhere and displacing T. mentagrophytes as the principal cause of tinea pedis.

Geographical Distribution - World-wide. Sporulating, non-fluffy isolates predominant in Pacific Islands and South Asia.

Appearance of Thallus - Typically a downy to fluffy white thallus which slowly develops deep venous-blood color on the underside as the culture matures. Usual European and American isolates produce dense white fluffy mycelium almost devoid of spores and may develop a greenish melanoid hue. Occasional strains produce macroaleuriospores in profusion. These tend to be less fluffy, slower growing, heaped up, and sometimes less intensely pigmented. Heaped-up relatively glabrous thalli may resemble T. violaceum. Sporulating strains are more typically isolated from tinea corporis, granulomatous lesions and tinea capitis than from usual tinea pedis, tinea cruris, and tinea manum. T. rubrum is distinguished from other red pigmented dermatophytes by its usually white fluffy or fuzzy surface and dark red non-diffusing pigment under the thallus and by its microscopic morphology. Plates III and IV.

Microscopic Morphology - The usual fluffy thallus of T. rubrum consists of long strands of hyphae with small, lateral, characteristically tear-shaped or peg-shaped microaleuriospores. Macroaleuriospores are absent or rare.

In sporulating strains macroaleuriospores may be abundant and characteristically narrow, long, and pencil-shaped, often developing directly at the ends of thick hyphae or attached together in a fashion resembling the macroaleuriospores of Epidermophyton floccosum. Microaleuriospores tend to be larger, clavate to round, and in small open clusters as well as along the hyphae. The production of microaleuriospores directly on macroaleuriospores is a rather common and characteristic feature in T. rubrum. Both hyphae and macroaleuriospores tend to break up into numerous arthrospores. Sporulating thalli must be distinguished microscopically from T. tonsurans and T. mentagrophytes by the form of the macro- and microaleuriospores.

T. soudanense-like reflexive branching is occasionally seen

Special Nutritional Requirements - None reported.

Variants - A very variable species. In general the various sporulating and non-sporulating forms are described above. To summarize: typical cultures of T. rubrum may vary in macroscopic appearance from fluffy through suede-like and folded (suggestive of T. tonsurans) to glabrous and heaped up (suggestive of T. violaceum) and in microscopic appearance from few to numerous peg-shaped microaleuriospores with or without macroaleuriospores to abundant macroaleuriospores with microaleuriospores tending to be egg-shaped and plump. An additional common variable feature is the tendency to produce arthrospores. Occasional strains produce little or no color and may be difficult to distinguish from pleomorphic T. mentagrophytes. In some strains and under alkaline conditions or poor aeration the undercolor of the thallus may be yellow rather than red. Rare strains produce a dark brown, diffusing melanoid pigment.

Perfect State - Not reported. Non-fertile ascocarps with peridial hyphae of the Arthroderma type may be produced in culture. All isolates so far tested against Arthroderma simii appear to be (-) mating type.

Special Media - Potato dextrose agar is useful to separate tinea pedis and tinea cruris strains of T. rubrum and T. mentagrophytes. Pigment formation is usually very intense on this medium and fluffy surface growth is reduced. Meat infusion agar will stimulate production of a few macroaleuriospores in many fluffy strains. T. rubrum grows well in absence of thiamine, serving to distinguish it from T. tonsurans and T. violaceum, and unlike T. megninii it does not require 1-histidine. T. rubrum may be distinguished from T. mentagrophytes by its failure to perforate hair in vitro and by the production of red pigment on corn meal dextrose agar. Urease activity weak except in granular variants.

Critical Characteristics - (1) Characteristics and pigment of thallus, (2) Tear-shaped microaleuriospores, (3) Characteristic macroaleuriospores, (4) Independent of thiamine and histidine, (5) Failure to perforate hair in vitro.

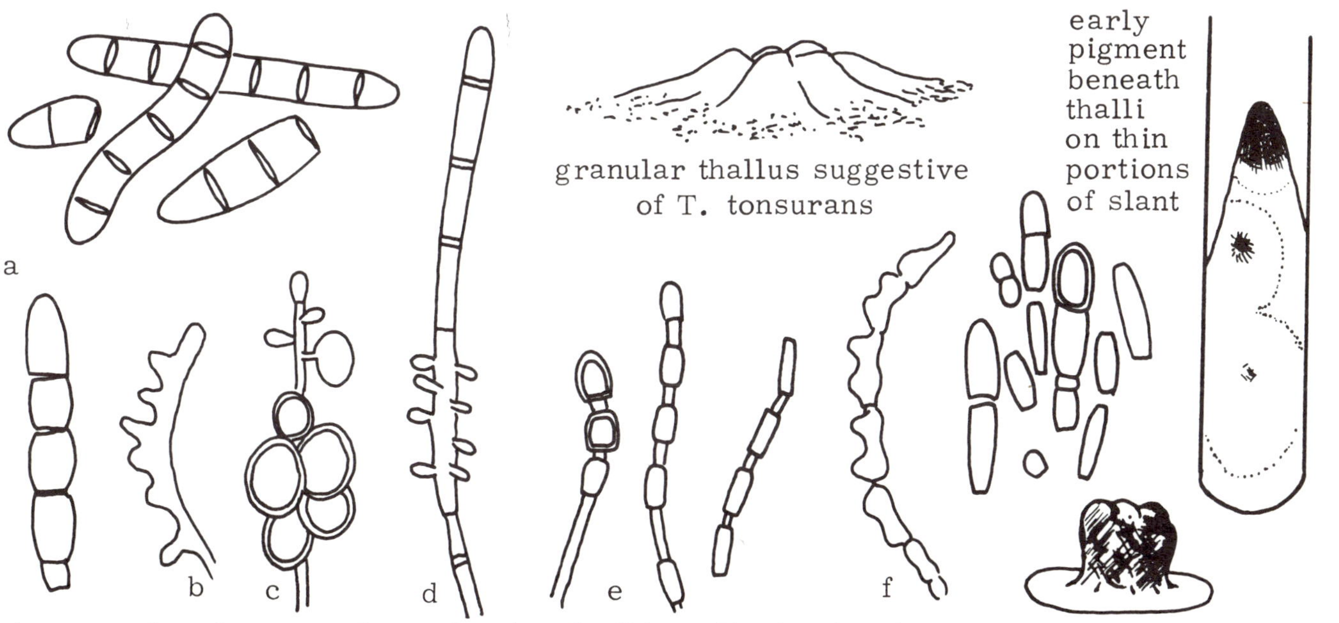

(a) macroaleuriospores (granular type), (b) pectinate structure, (c) enlarged microaleuriospores and chlamydospores, (d) macroaleuriospores bearing lateral microaleuriospores, (e) arthroaleuriospores, (f) peridial hypha from sterile ascocarp.

microscopic features and thallus of glabrous (rodhainii) variant

Identification of Trichophyton tonsurans

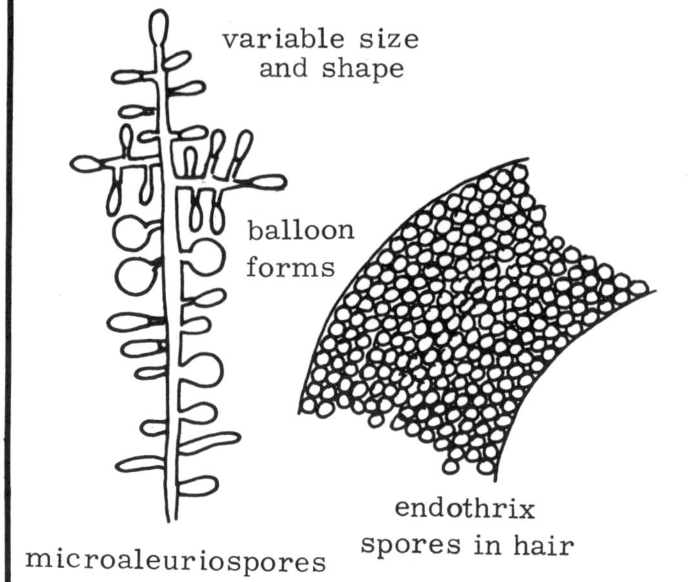

Invasion of Hair - Abundant endothrix; sporulating in chains inside the hair shaft causes the hair to burst, crumble and curl, producing a black dot or chicken skin effect on the scalp. No fluorescence. Obtain hair for examination by scraping black dot, not plucking.

Clinical Disease - Primarily a scalp ringworm, but frequently causes tinea corporis, and occasionally onychomycosis and tinea pedis. May occur in older women. Usually non-inflammatory. Kerion may occur, however.

Epidemiology - Infects only man. Contagious.

Geographical Distribution - World-wide. Probably originally described as an Old World species, now endemic and particularly abundant in Mexico and other Latin American countries and has become very prevalent in the United States and Canada following Latin immigrations.

Appearance of Thallus - The mahogany red form on first isolation often a flat, somewhat powdery, yellowish thallus with more or less of a mahogany red undercolor. Develops into a folded thallus with a suede-like surface which varies from cream-white to greyish or brownish buff, sometimes with pink tints. Undersurface of colony may be reddish brown and dark pigment may diffuse into the medium. The sulfureum form on first isolation a relatively less powdery, pale to deep yellow thallus which develops a suede-like surface which varies from clear yellow to grey-white. Relatively colorless forms also occur. Plates III and IV.

Microscopic Morphology - The microaleuriospores are the most diagnostic feature. They are usually abundant and of large or variable size, tear-drop or club-shaped on open branching clusters or thickened terminal hyphae. A characteristic feature is the tendency of individual microaleuriospores to enlarge resulting in clavate or balloon forms. Clustered balloon forms also seen occasionally in T. rubrum and T. mentagrophytes. Macroaleuriospores often are somewhat thick walled, are usually less perfectly formed than T. mentagrophytes, and blunter than T. rubrum. Arthrospores frequent. May have spiral coils. Absence of elongated macroaleuriospores distinguishes T. tonsurans from sporulating forms of T. rubrum.

Special Nutritional Requirements - Like T. violaceum, T. tonsurans grows better if thiamine is available.

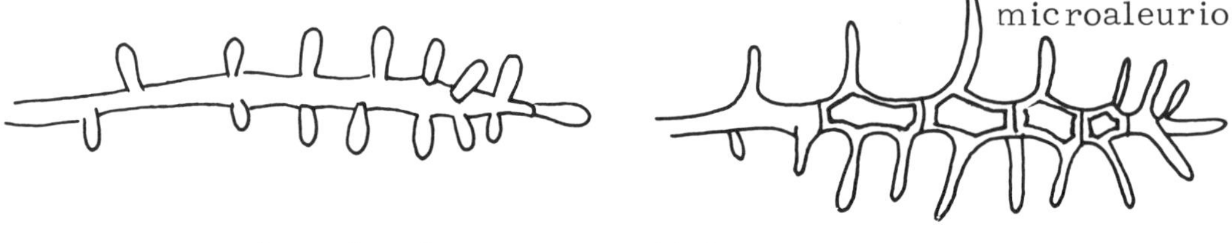

filiform microaleuriospores

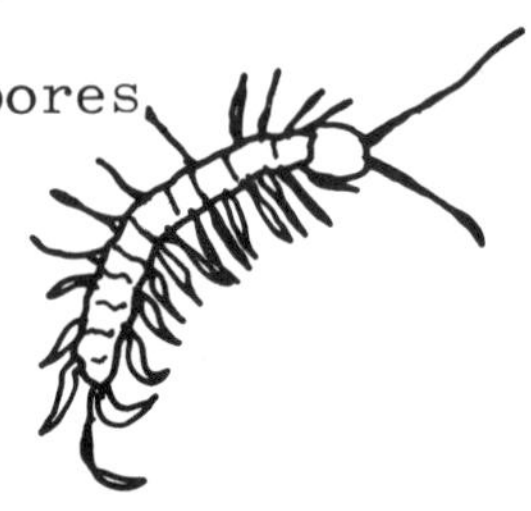

microaleuriospores on thickened hyphae

Trichophyton tonsurans - Cont.

Variants - The sulfureum variety may predominate in certain localities and superficially may resemble Epidermophyton floccosum. Differently folding types were formerly classed as different species (crateriforme, cerebriforme, plicatile, etc.).

Perfect State - Not reported.

Special Media - The partial requirement of T. tonsurans for thiamine may be used to separate it from T. mentagrophytes, T. rubrum and T. megninii. See page 48.

Critical Characteristics - (1) Characteristic microaleuriospores and total microscopic morphology, (2) Colony form, (3) Thiamine requirement.

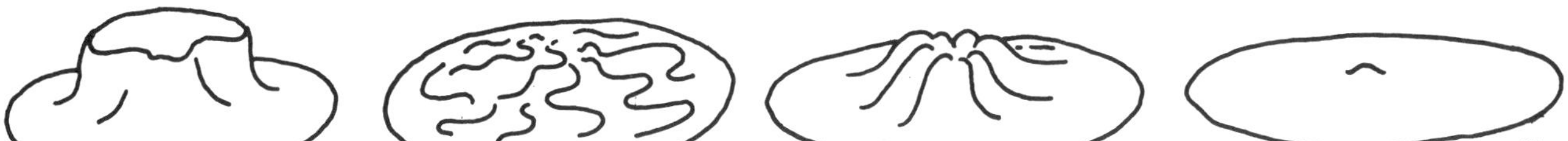

flat

crateriforme cerebriforme plicatile Types of Folding of Thallus Surface

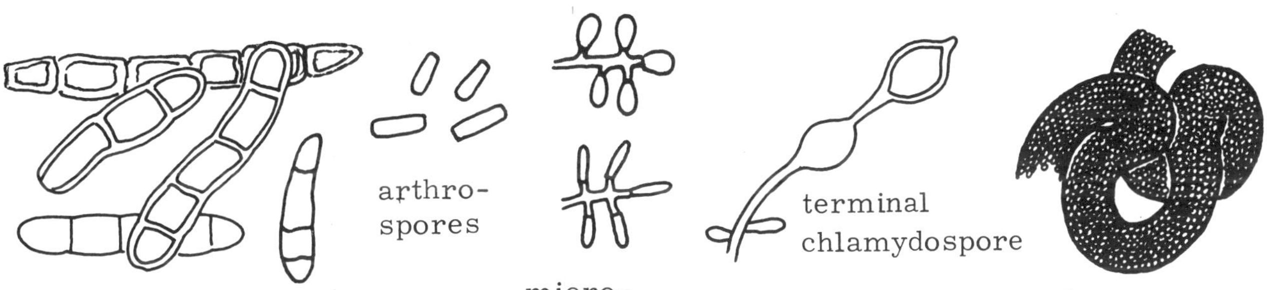

macroaleuriospores micro-aleuriospores hair coiled in stratum corneum (black dot)

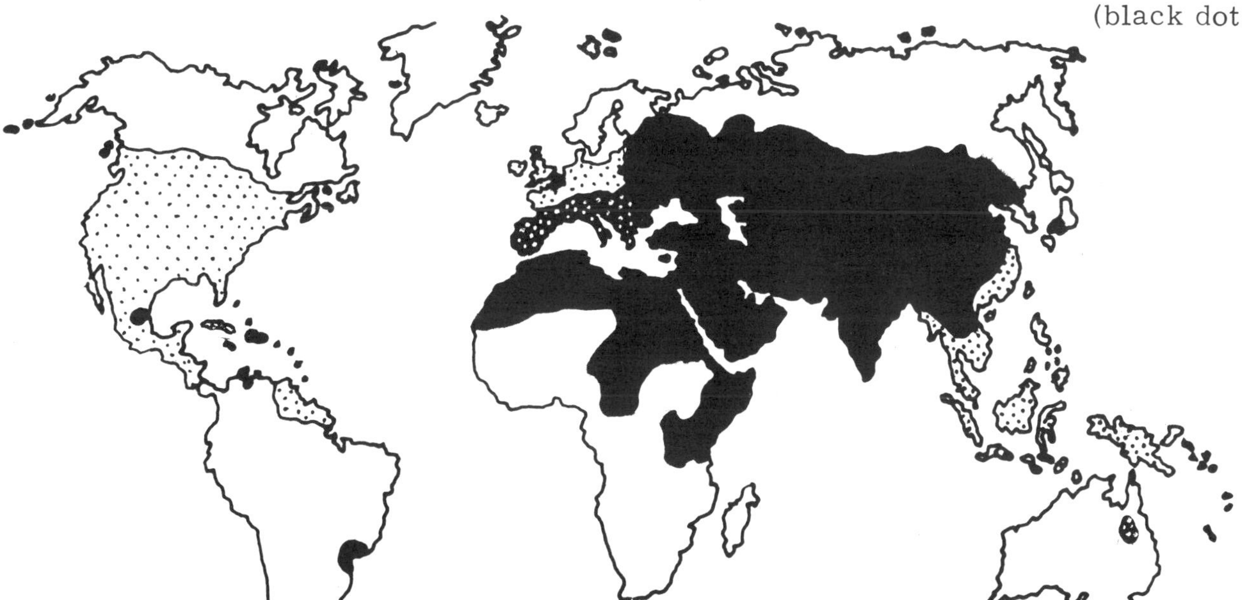

Major distribution of endothrix tinea capitis I (see also page 57)

T. tonsurans ▒ T. violaceum ■

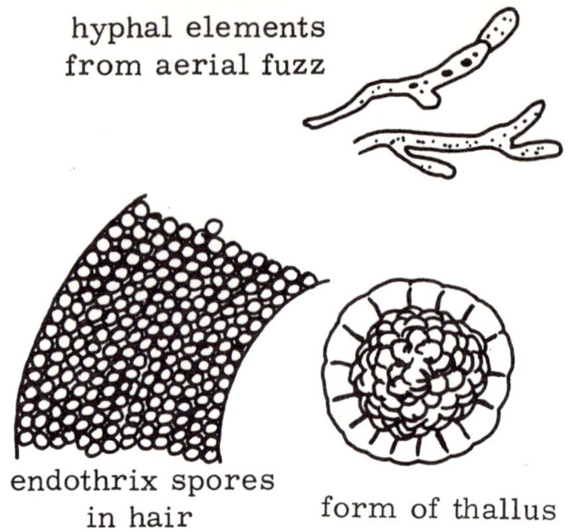

Identification of Trichophyton violaceum

Invasion of Hair - Identical to that seen with T. tonsurans.

Clinical Disease - Usually similar to that seen with T. tonsurans, probably a greater frequency of tinea corporis, onychomycosis, inflammatory response, bald patches and scarring. May produce favus-like crusts.

Epidemiology - Similar to T. tonsurans.

Geographical Distribution - One of the most important causes of scalp ringworm, particularly in the Near East, Eastern Europe, Russia and North Africa. Relatively uncommon in North America north of Mexico, although institutional epidemics may occur. Locally endemic in Latin America. Map page 53.

Appearance of Thallus - When first isolated usually a waxy, wrinkled, heaped up or verrucous thallus which turns deep purplish-red. This form is very difficult to keep in subculture and thalli tend to rapidly become more downy, paler in color and develop pale sectors. Stock cultures rapidly die when stored in the refrigerator. Plate III.

Microscopic Morphology - Typically a tortuous tangle of branched hyphae (containing cytoplasmic granules) with no aleuriospores. The sparse aerial hyphae may have thickened elements that resemble macroaleuriospores of the T. rubrum type. Pyriform microaleuriospores have been observed on enriched media and rarely clavate macroaleuriospores.

Special Nutritional Requirements - All strains of T. violaceum like T. tonsurans are partially dependent on thiamine. Growth in the absence of thiamine is minimal.

Variants - Because of sectoring and pleomorphism no two isolates remain exactly alike. Non-pigmented glabrous isolates were previously called T. glabrum.

Perfect State - Not reported.

Special Media - Demonstration of partial requirement for thiamine may be necessary to distinguish T. violaceum from T. gourvilii, T. rubrum, and other dermatophytes of similar morphology.

Critical Characteristics - (1) Purplish glabrous thallus, (2) Thiamine requirement, (3) Microscopic morphology, (4) Endothrix non-fluorescent hair invasion.

macro- and microaleuriospores
produced in presence of thiamine

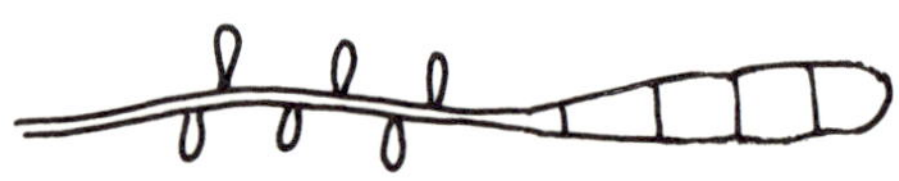

Reference: "Trichophyton violaceum" by P. Pinotti, Edizione Minerva Medica, 1962.

Identification of Trichophyton gourvilii

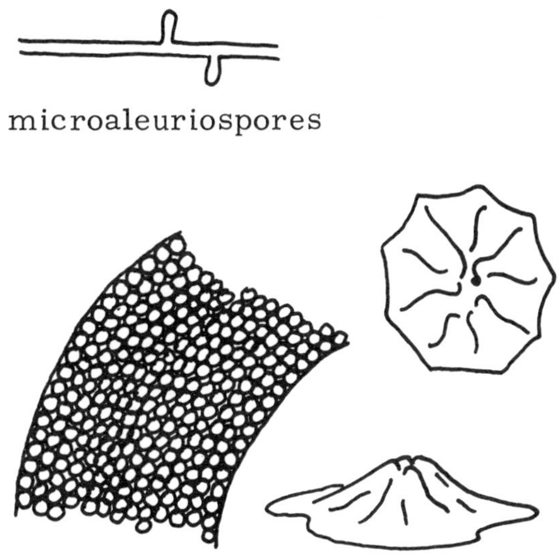

microaleuriospores

endothrix spores in hair

form of thallus

Invasion of Hair - Endothrix as in T. tonsurans and T. violaceum.

Clinical Disease - Similar to T. tonsurans and T. violaceum.

Epidemiology - Similar to T. tonsurans and T. violaceum.

Geographical Distribution - Parts of West Africa north of the Congo (Algeria, Chad, Ivory Coast, French Sudan, Republic of the Congo, Senegal, Togo, Upper Volta). Map Page 57.

Appearance of Thallus - A folded and heaped up waxy thallus which tends on transfer to become spreading and satiny with a lavender-pink to garnet-red color. A mollasses brown color may diffuse into the medium. Plate III.

Microscopic Morphology - Microaleuriospores and macroaleuriospores of the Trichophyton type are usually present.

Special Nutritional Requirements - None known.

Variants - There seems a possibility of confusing T. gourvilii, T. megninii, T. rubrum, T. violaceum, and T. soudanense (violet form) in Europe and Africa. All these species have been reported to produce endothrix tinea capitis.

Perfect State - Not described.

Special Media - Growth in the absence of thiamine and histidine serves to distinguish the species from T. violaceum and T. megninii respectively.

Critical Characteristics - (1) Appearance of thallus, (2) Lack of thiamine requirement, (3) Geographical distribution, (4) Presence of microaleuriospores and macroaleuriospores, (5) Endothrix hair invasion.

References:

Catanei, A., 1933. Description de Trichophyton gourvili n. sp., Agent D'une Teigne de L'homme, Bull. Soc. Path. exot., 26:377-381.

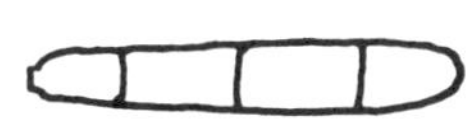

macroaleuriospore

Identification of Trichophyton soudanense

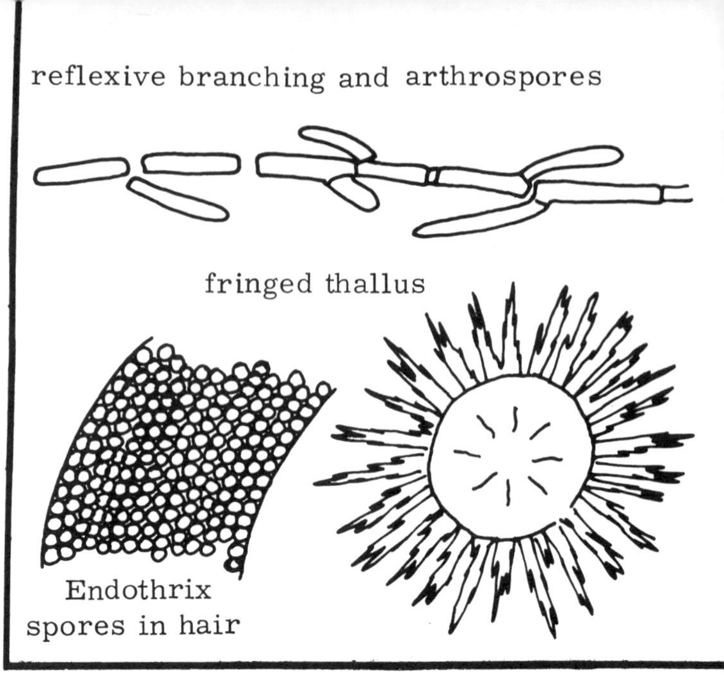

Invasion of Hair - Sporulation is endothrix as in T. tonsurans and T. violaceum.

Clinical Disease - Principally a cause of tinea capitis and associated tinea corporis. Probably more frequently inflammatory than infections with T. yaoundei.

Epidemiology - There are five agents of endothrix tinea capitis in Africa. This is one of the commoner and widespread species. Infections of the scalp with two or more species of dermatophytes is not uncommon in African Negro children.

Geographical Distribution - Widespread in Africa. Reported principally from West Africa (Algeria to Angola and into the Congo). Appearing in Great Britain and other countries receiving African immigrants. Occasional reports from the United States from Negro and white patients without clue to origin. Has similarly been isolated from child in Brazil.

Appearance of Thallus - A slow-growing, flat to folded, suede-like, yellow, dried apricot-colored thallus, often with a submerged and fringed (eyelash) border. Develops pleomorphism readily. Does not survive refrigeration. Plate III.

Microscopic Morphology - Mycelia usually characterized by breaking up into segments or arthrospores and backward growing (reflexive) or right angle branching, forming bush-like bundles which account for the fringes. Delicate Trichophyton type pyriform microconidia may occur along the hyphae, reported as abundant on Dubos media, but are not in themselves diagnostic.

Special Nutritional Requirements - Will not grow on ammonium nitrate or histidine as nitrogen source. Is not stimulated by thiamine.

Variants - Mutants with a purplish color on Sabouraud agar may be produced on subculture.

Perfect State - Not known.

Special Media - Not ordinarily required. Colony dark on Lowenstein's egg medium and Dubos medium as compared to M. ferrugineum.*

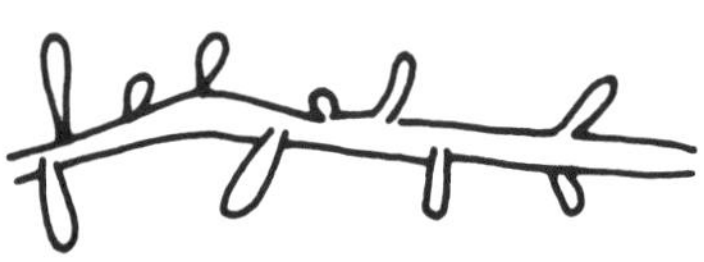

microaleuriospores

* Vanbreuseghem, R. and Zana, R., 1963. Ann. Soc. Belge Med. Trop., 43:259-270. (Lowenstein - Jensen and Dubois are standard bacteriological media for Mycobacteria and available commercially in prepared form)

Trichophyton soudanense - Cont.

Critical Characteristics - (1) Thallus appearance, (2) Microscopic morphology, (3) Endothrix hair invasion.

References:

Rippon, J.W. and Medenica, M., 1964. Isolation of Trichophyton soudanense in the United States, Sabouraudia, 3:301-302.

Johnson, J.A. and Rosenthal, S.A., 1968. Superficial Cutaneous Infection with Trichophyton soudanense, Arch. Derm., 97:428-431.

Vanbreuseghem, R., 1968. Trichophyton soudanense In and Outside Africa, Brit. J. Dermat., 80:140-148.

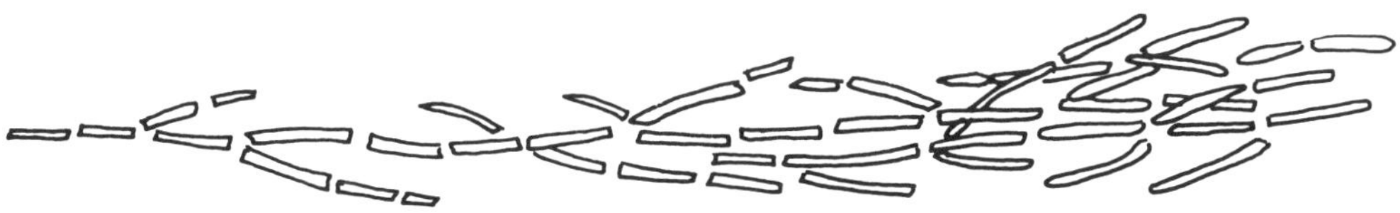

bundles of arthrospores with reflexive branching

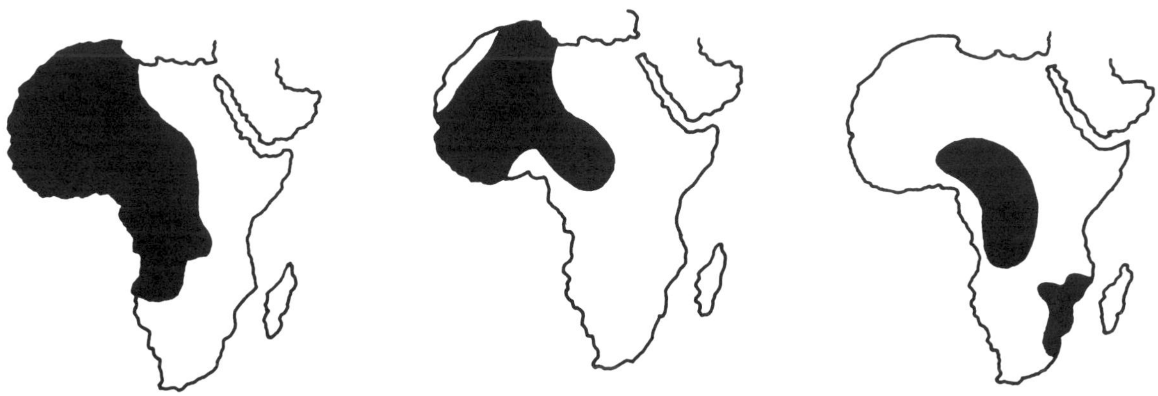

T. soudanense　　T. gourvilii　　T. yaoundei

distribution of endothrix tinea capitis II (see also page 53)

Identification of Trichophyton yaoundei

Invasion of Hair - Sporulation is endothrix as in T. tonsurans and T. violaceum.

Clinical Disease - Primarily a cause of tinea capitis similar to that seen with T. tonsurans and T. violaceum.

Epidemiology - A locally common native endothrix species in Equatorial Africa (Mozambique and Republic of the Congo) where tinea capitis caused by M. audouinii, M. ferrugineum, T. violaceum, T. soudanense and the present species is rampant.

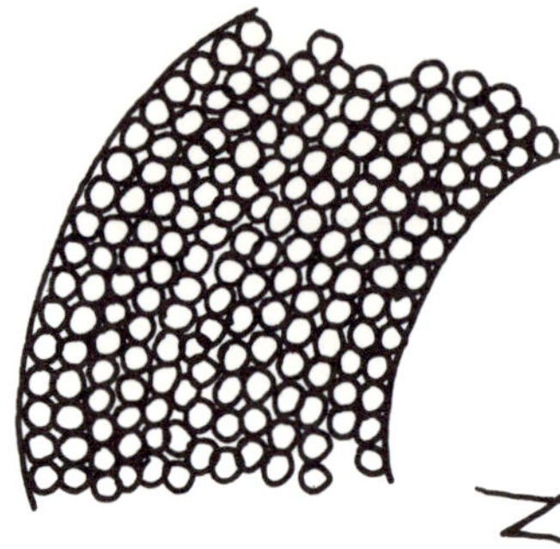

endothrix spores in hair

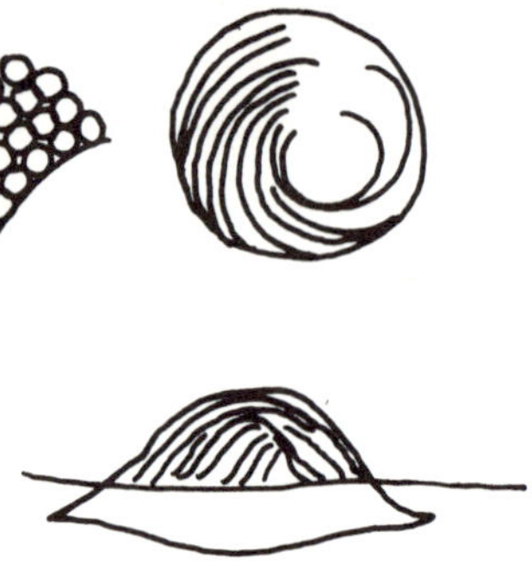

form of thallus

Geographical Distribution - To date isolated from the Cameroon and Congo, and other African countries. One report from the British Isles in a migrant from Africa. Map page 57.

Appearance of Thallus - Usually an extremely glabrous, almost wet looking, heaped-up or subsurface, slow growing thallus which sooner or later turns a deep tan or chocolate brown color which diffuses into the media. Strains in stock cultivation may lose this characteristic brown color. Plate III.

Microscopic Morphology - Trichophyton type pyriform microaleuriospores are rare. Typical macroaleuriospores are not formed. The short aerial hyphae may contain chlamydospore elements similar to those seen in T. violaceum.

Special Nutritional Requirements - None observed.

Variants - Like T. violaceum, T. yaoundei has a marked tendency to sector and undergo pleomorphic change, so that no two isolates or cultures remain quite alike.

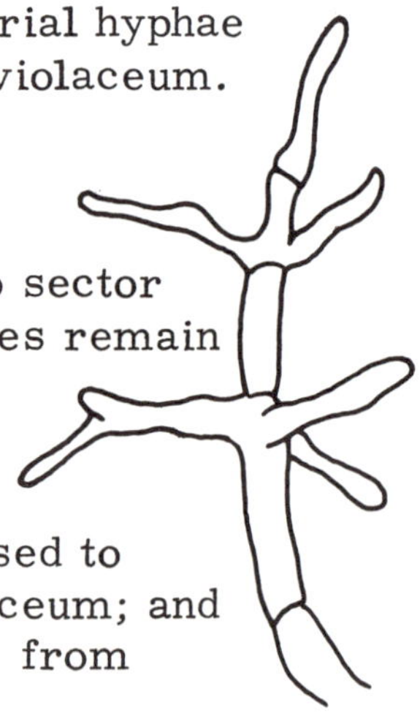

mycelial feature

Perfect State - Not known.

Special Media - The absence of a requirement for thiamine may be used to separate from T. verrucosum and the glabrum variety of T. violaceum; and ability to grow on NH_4NO_3 or histidine as only source of nitrogen, from T. soudanense.

Critical Characteristics - (1) Appearance of thallus, (2) Endothrix hair invasion, (3) Geographical distribution, (4) Lack of requirement for thiamine.

Reference:

Georg, L.K., Doupagne, P., Pattyn, S.R. and Neves, H., 1963. Trichophyton yaoundei, A Dermatophyte Indigenous to Africa, J. Invest. Derm., 41:19-24.

Identification of Trichophyton schoenleinii

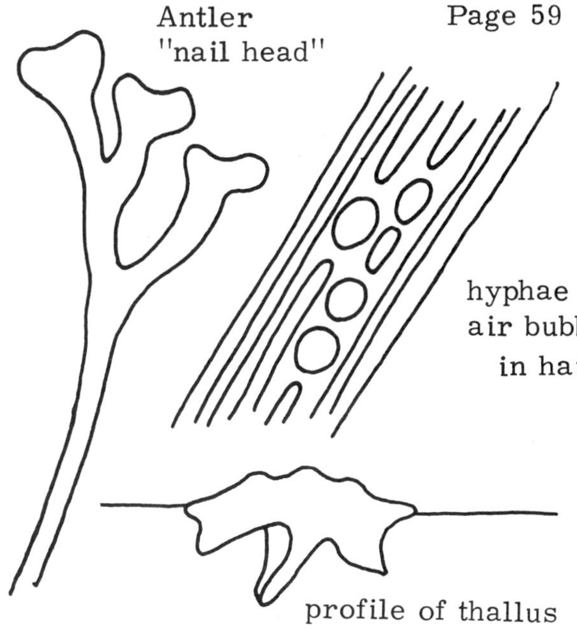

Invasion of Hair - Invasion of hair with T. schoenleinii is characteristic. Within the hair, hyphae and air spaces occupied by degenerate hyphae are seen. Arthrospores are few or absent. Infected hairs remain intact, often an inch or more long and frequently exhibit a dull bluish-white fluorescence. In typical favus, elevated, yellowish, cup-like crusts or mats of hyphae (scutula or godets) occur in the hair follicles of the scalp and body. Similar crusts are occasionally seen with M. gypseum in mouse favus in man due to T. mentagrophytes and rarely with T. violaceum.

Clinical Disease - The typical and usual cause of favus, a chronic, scarring form of tinea capitis distinguished by the formation of scutula, crusts, scarring, atrophy and permanent hair loss. T. schoenleinii also produces a type of scaling tinea capitis which can be mistaken for non-mycotic conditions such as dandruff, seborrhea, tinea amiantacea, or impetigo. Tinea corporis, often with scutula and onychomycosis are not infrequent. Fatal brain abscess has been reported.

Epidemiology - An anthropophilic infection which because of its disfiguring effects constitutes a most serious form of dermatophyte infection.

Geographical Distribution - Widespread in Eurasia and North Africa where it shares with T. violaceum a place of predominance among the agents of tinea capitis. The disease is less frequent in the Western Hemisphere although endemic foci occur. These may be confined to the members of a single family or clan.

Appearance of Thallus - A waxy to slightly downy white or off-white thallus, with a heaped or convoluted surface resembling beeswax, plaster of paris, or raw pie crust. New isolates may grow out yeast-like in consistency, and microscopically resemble the yeast phase of Blastomyces dermatiditis. Strains in laboratory cultivation tend to become more and more downy and spreading. Thalli characteristically grow rather deep into the agar and often split the medium. Some strains produce mainly subsurface growth. Plate III.

Microscopic Morphology - Macro- and microaleuriospores are virtually never seen. Characteristic antler-like hyphae are produced in the subsurface growth. Antler-like terminal branching is common in many slow growing dermatophyte thalli, but the swollen hyphal tips (nail-head hyphae) are not frequently seen except in T. schoenleinii. (See also T. verrucosum and T. concentricum). Initial outgrowth from clinical material may consist of spherical yeast-like arthrospores.

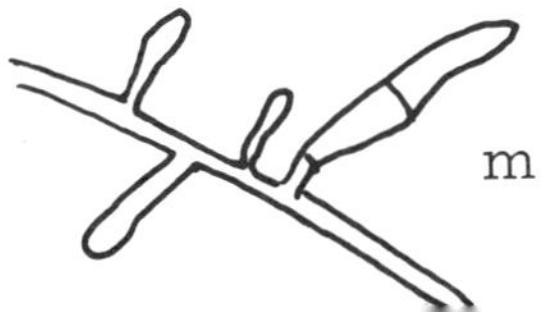

Trichophyton schoenleinii - Cont.

Special Nutritional Requirements - None known.

Variants - Thalli in cultivation vary from glabrous and heaped to silky, downy and spreading, and from white to grey-brown in color.

Perfect State - Not known.

Special Media - Growth on medium without thiamine distinguishes this species from T. verrucosum, T. violaceum and many strains of T. concentricum.

Critical Characteristics - (1) Morphology of thallus and favic type antler hyphae, (2) Clinical lesions and hair invasion, (3) Growth in absence of thiamine.

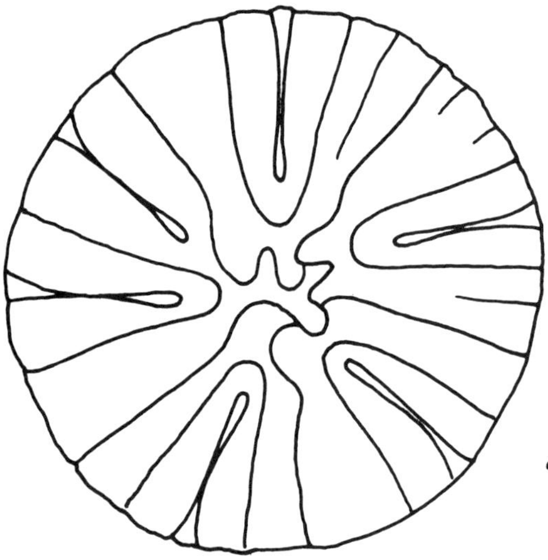

thallus in laboratory culture

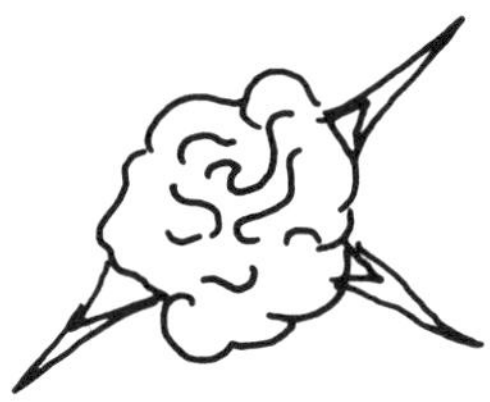

thallus of freshly isolated strain

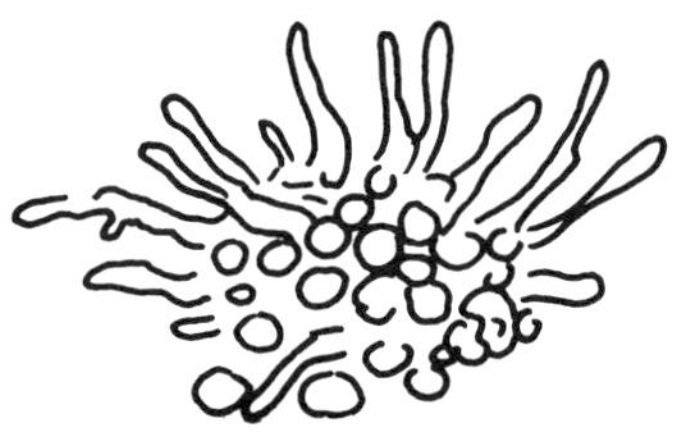

portion of scutula

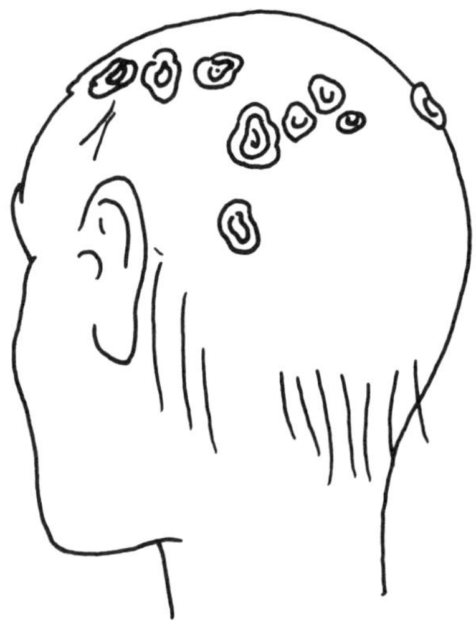

favus showing alopecia and scutula

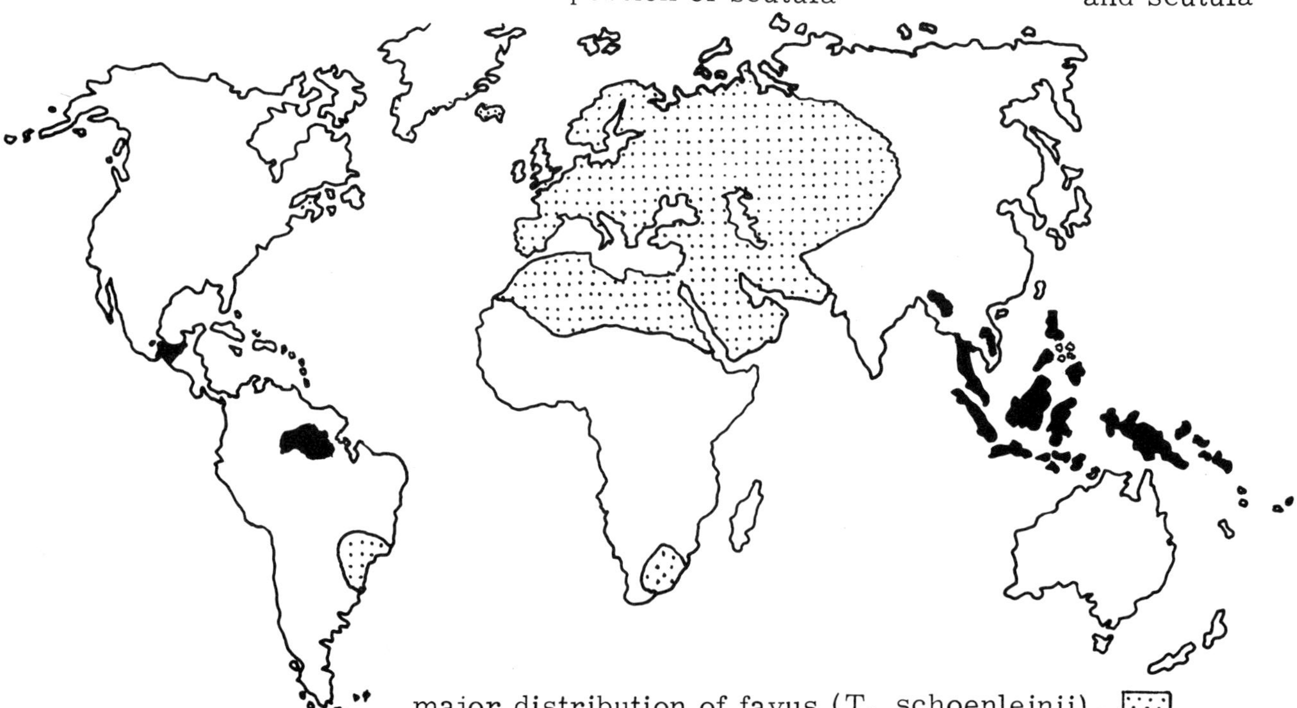

major distribution of favus (T. schoenleinii)
and tinea imbricata (T. concentricum)

Identification of Trichophyton concentricum

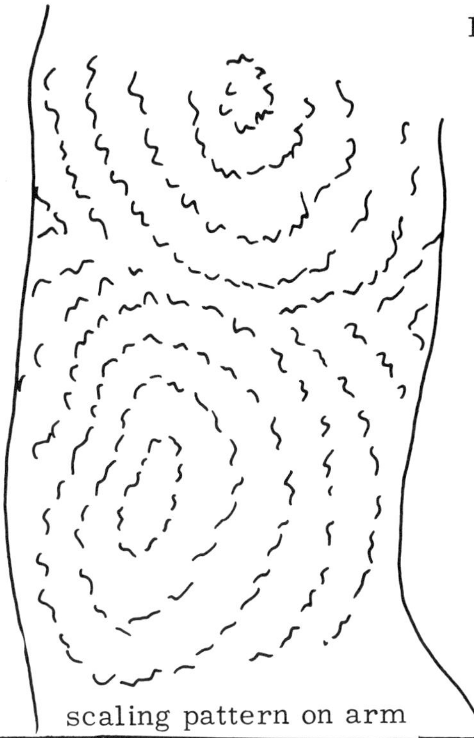

scaling pattern on arm

Invasion of Hair - Not known to invade hair.

Clinical Disease - Cause of tinea imbricata (tokelau) a form of tinea corporis in which concentric rings of scaling are produced on the skin. The lesions may develop to cover the entire body with gyrate patterns or be more or less lichenified due to scratching. Usually intensely pruritic.

Epidemiology - An anthropophilic species involving native peoples. Rare among Europeans.

Geographical Distribution - The major endemic area is the South Pacific Islands and adjacent mainland. Present in aboriginal populations in the interior of South Asia (Vietnamese highlands, etc.). Also endemic in Guatemala, Southern Mexico, and central Brazil among forest Indians. Map page 60.

Appearance of Thallus - A white, honey to brown colored, or orange-brown, much folded, slow growing thallus, which tends to become slightly velvety in stock culture. Usually somewhat more glabrous, densely convoluted and browner than T. schoenleinii which it closely resembles. Plate III.

Microscopic Morphology - Tangled and branching hyphae without micro-or macro-aleuriospores. Terminal branching but usually without the swollen nail-head hyphae typical of T. schoenleinii.

Special Nutritional Requirements - Many but not all strains are stimulated by thiamine.

Variants - Varies from whitish to brown. A slightly downy flat (indicum) variant may be isolated.

Perfect State - Not known.

Special Media - Slight response to thiamine in about 50% of isolates may be used as an aid in distinguishing some strains from T. schoenleinii and T. verrucosum with which it has been confused.

Critical Characteristics - (1) Clinical disease, (2) Morphology of thallus, (3) Local geographical distribution, (4) Frequent slight response to thiamine.

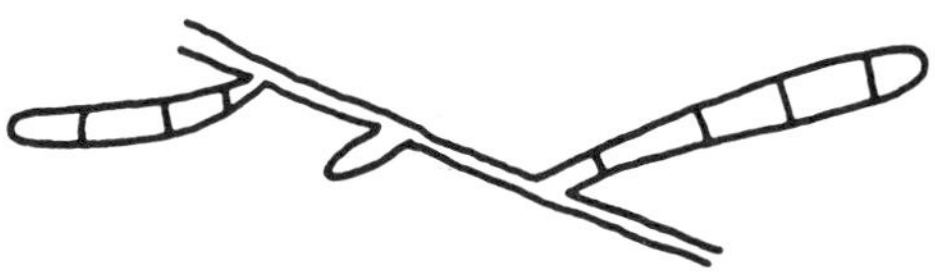

Lateral macroconidia on bean pod agar (Ahearn, U. of Miami)

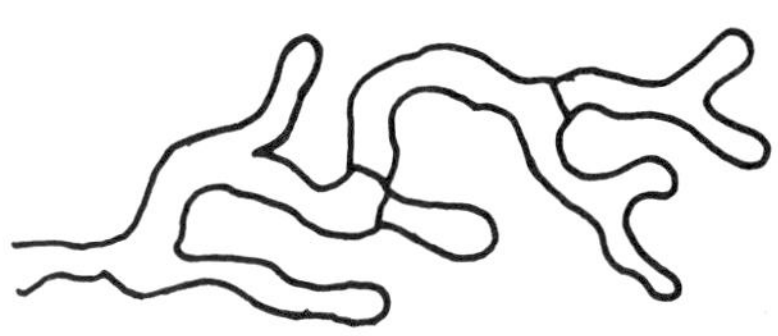

mycelial feature

Identification of <u>Epidermophyton floccosum</u>

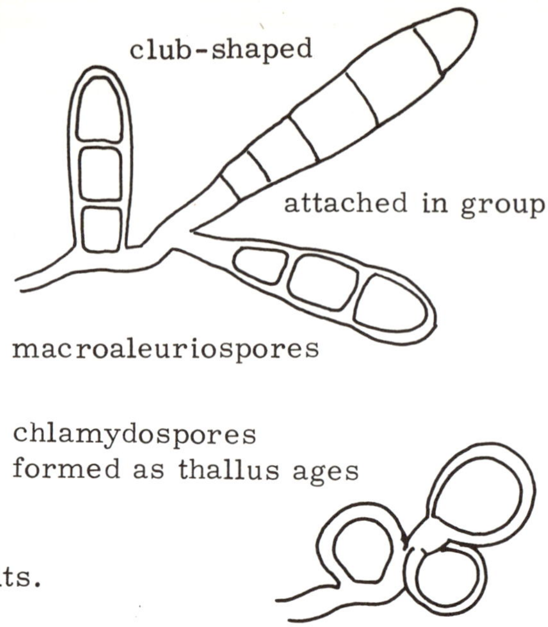

Invasion of Hair - Not known to invade hair.

Clinical Disease - Regularly responsible for a small percentage of tinea cruris, tinea pedis, tinea corporis and onychomycosis. Generalized infections have been reported.

Epidemiology - With very rare exceptions, infects only man. May become epidemic among personnel using common shower and gym facilities. Common cause of groin infections in military recruits.

Geographical Distribution - World-wide.

Appearance of Thallus - Primary isolates are often grainy, lumpy and sparse, and of a yellow-mustard to olive-grey color. On subculture typically a folded thallus with the fuzzy texture of suede. Olive-green tint or khaki color of thallus a hall mark. Regularly develops white tufts of pleomorphism; pleomorphic thalli become white and densely fluffy. The colonies are difficult to maintain since they do not survive refrigeration. Plates III and IV.

Microscopic Morphology - Characteristic blunt, club-shaped macroaleuriospores attached together in groups are best seen in early stages of colony. Macroaleuriospores undergo transformation into chlamydospores in older colonies. No microaleuriospores are formed. Spiral coils are sometimes seen but are not diagnostic.

Special Nutritional Requirements - None reported.

Variants - Isolates vary from olive-grey to yellowish-olive. Macroaleuriospores vary from blunt to long clubs.

Perfect State - Not reported.

Special Media - None required.

Critical Characteristics - (1) Characteristic macroaleuriospores, (2) No microaleuriospores, (3) Appearance of thallus.

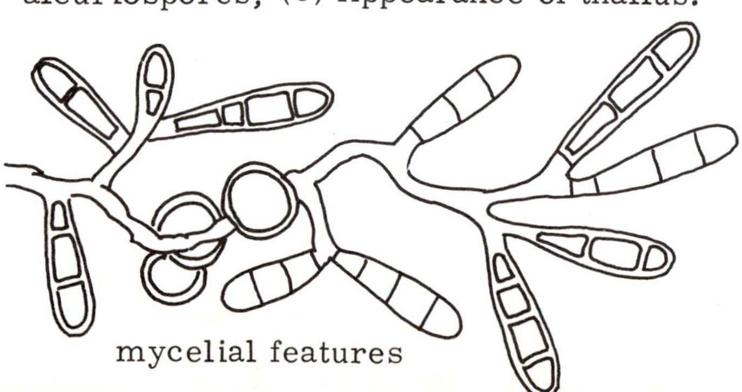

mycelial features

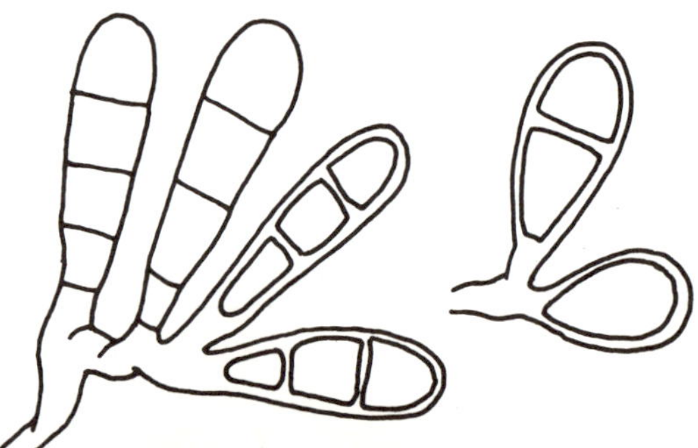

macroaleuriospore shapes

Additional Species of Microsporum

Identification of Microsporum boullardi

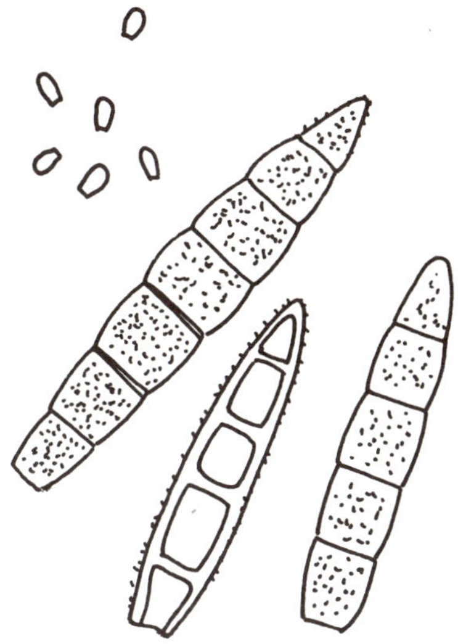

Appearance of Thallus - Similar to M. fulvum, but somewhat more powdery. Pink-buff, with apple red to purplish undercolor.

Microscopic Morphology - The macroaleuriospores resemble those of strains of M. fulvum which produce bullet-shaped macroaleuriospores, except that they are larger, longer, and have thicker walls. As compared to M. racemosum and M. praecox, the macroaleuriospores of M. boullardi are less than 60 microns long and are more cylindrical, bullet-shaped, or cigar-shaped, and have more closely spaced cells. Clavate microaleuriospores are usually abundant.

Occurrence - Isolated from soil in Conakry, Africa.

Comment - M. boullardi is difficult to separate from some strains of M. fulvum, unless typical large macroaleuriospores are present. Does not form ascospores with N. fulva.

Critical Characteristics - (1) Macroaleuriospores, (2) Appearance of thallus, (3) Failure to produce ascospores with N. fulva.

References:

Dominik, T. and Majchrowicz, I., 1965. Second Contribution to the Knowledge of Keratinolytic and Keratinophilic Soil Fungi in the Region of Szczecin. Ecologia Polska-Ser. A., 13:415-447.

Dominik, T. and Majchrowicz, I., 1966. Some New Species of Fungi from the Soil of Conakry. Mycopathologia, 28:209-219.

Additional Species of Microsporum

Identification of Microsporum praecox

Appearance of Thallus - Similar to M. gypseum. Powdery buff with yellow-orange undersurface.

Microscopic Morphology - The macroaleuriospores, although thin-walled like M. gypseum, are long, narrow, and lanceolate in profile, exceeding 60 microns in length and 9 microns in width, with 6 to 9 cells. Compared to M. racemosum the macroaleuriospores are more uniform in size.

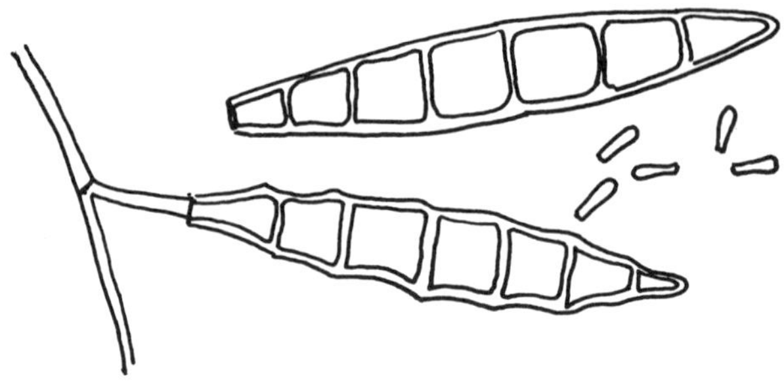

macro- and microaleuriospores

Occurrence - Isolated from a pustular vesicular ringworm lesion on the wrist in France.

Critical Characteristics - (1) Macroaleuriospores, (2) Appearance of thallus, (3) Failure to produce ascospores with Nannizzia gypsea, incurvata or fulva.

References:

Rivalier, E., 1953. Description de Sabouraudites praecox nova Species Suivie de Remarques Sur le Genre Sabouraudites, Ann. de Inst. Pasteur 86: 276-284.

Segretain, G., 1962. Some New or Infrequent Fungous Pathogens, Chapter IV in "Fungi and Fungous Diseases", Dalldorf, G., ed. C.C. Thomas, USA, pages 33-35.

Identification of Microsporum racemosum

Appearance of Thallus - Spreads very rapidly over the agar surface. The fastest growing dermatophyte. Surface of thallus powdery cream-white, becoming more or less stained with grape-red. Undersurface grape-red.

micro- and macroaleuriospores

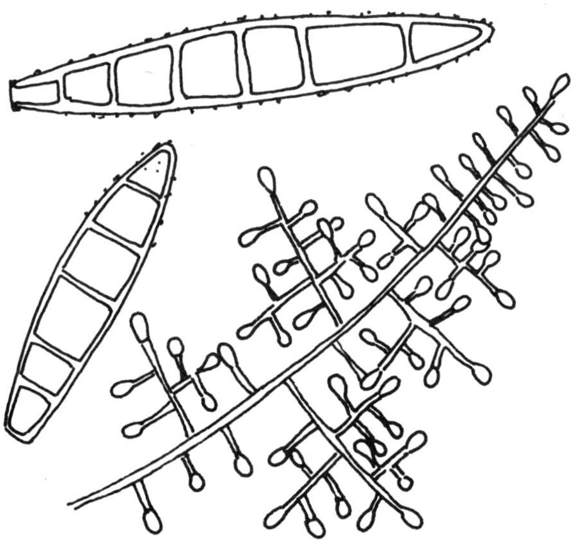

Microscopic Morphology - Macroaleuriospores becoming largest of any of the thin-walled species of Microsporum, but normally ranging in size from that of M. gypseum size, with 5 cells, to over 60μ long, spindle-shaped, and with up to 10 cells. The macroaleuriospores are tapered, not bullet-shaped as in M. boullardi. The microaleuriospores are distinctive. They are club-shaped, mostly stalked, and are in large, wand-like clusters or racemes.

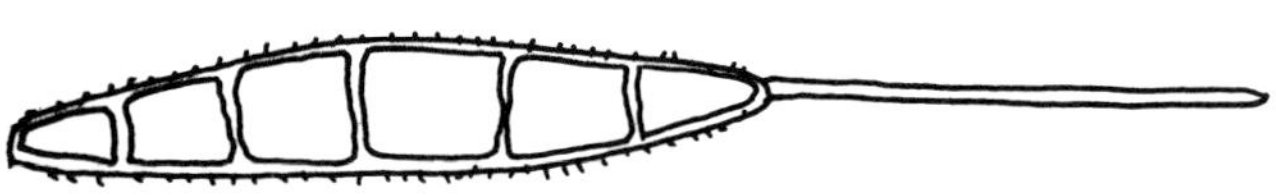

Macroaleuriospores frequently have terminal filaments.

Microsporum racemosum - Cont.

Occurrence - Isolated from soil in South America and Romania, probably world-wide. Potentially pathogenic on the basis of experimental lesions. Optimum growth at 23 - 28°C. Poor growth at 37°C.

Comment - M. racemosum and M. vanbreuseghemii are the only geophilic Microsporum species with a flat, initially cream-colored powdery surface. Report of ascigerous state in press (Mycologia 62, No. 4, 1970).

Critical Characteristics - (1) Appearance of thallus, (2) Macroaleuriospores, (3) Microaleuriospores.

Reference:

Borelli, D., 1965. Microsporum racemosum nova Species, Acta. Méd. Venez. 12:148-151.

Alteras, I. and Evolceanu, R., 1969. First Isolation of Microsporum racemosum Dante Borelli 1965 from Romanian Soil (New Data on its Pathogenic Properties), Mykosen 12:223-230.

Appearance of Microsporum amazonicum

Morphology of Thallus - Fluffy to heavily powdery, with a distinctive grey-olive buff color which is different from any other dermatophyte or related fungus except Ctenomyces serratus.

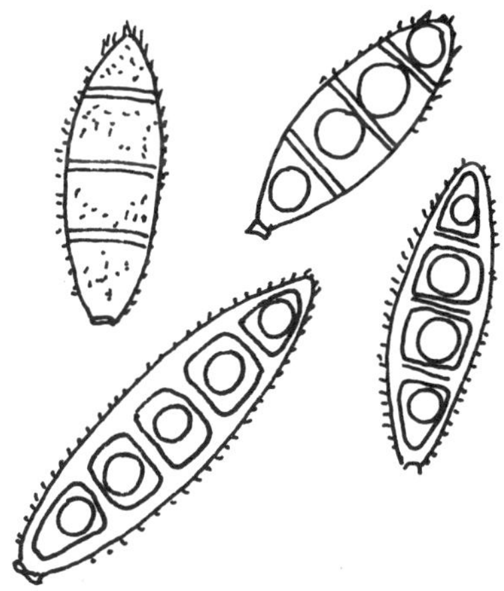

macroaleuriospores

Microscopic Morphology - The macroaleuriospores are characteristic. Symmetrical and spindle-shaped, with up to 7 or 8 cells, they have the following distinctive features: (1) predominantly four cells only, (2) a very small attachment scar, (3) rather thick walls and septa, (4) a large, oil droplet-like inclusion in each cell, and (5) a rather bristly echinulate surface. Smaller macroaleuriospores of M. gypseum may have these features.

Occurrence - Two isolates from apparently normal hairs of native rats (Oryzymys sp.) in Brazil. Grows poorly at 35°C, not at all at 37°C, and optimally from 23 - 28°C.

Critical Characteristics - (1) Macroaleuriospores, (2) Appearance of the thallus.

Reference:

Moraes, M., Borelli, D., and Feo, M., 1967. Microsporum amazonicum nova. Species. Medicinia Cutanea 11·281-286.

Additional Species of Trichophyton

Identification of Trichophyton phaseoliforme

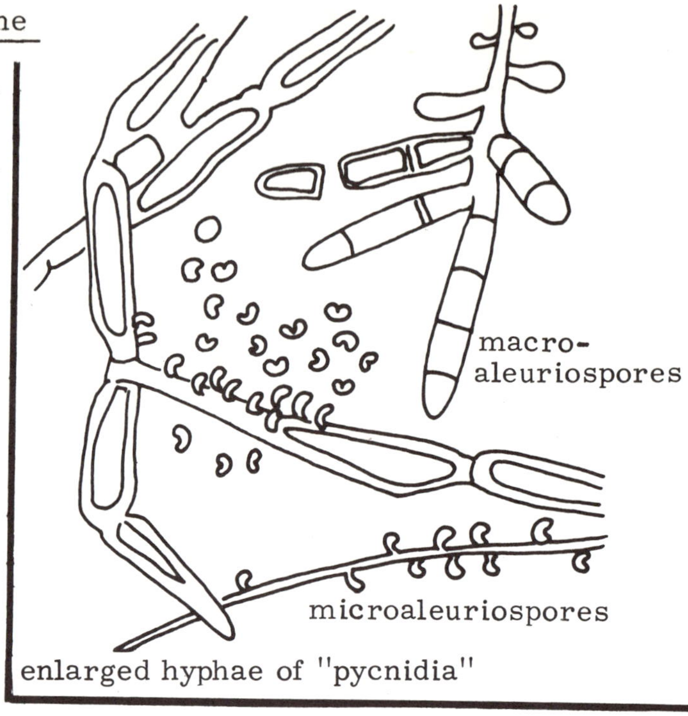

Appearance of Thallus - A powdery, white to bright cinnamon thallus which develops white or ivory colored spherical ascocarp-like structures on the surface.

Microscopic Morphology - The microaleuriospores are characteristically curved, cashew-nut shaped, and are borne laterally on the vegetative hyphae and in large numbers on thickened and enlarged hyphae in the ascocarp-like structures (pycnidia). The enlarged hyphae are smooth-surfaced and angular and do not resemble the peridial hyphae of Arthroderma and Nannizzia (which sometimes form sterile ascocarps or pycnidia-like structures in other dermatophytes). Cylindrical macroaleuriospores are produced in terminal clusters and are suggestive of T. terrestre and T. gloriae. One celled forms may be curved and intermediate with the microaleuriospores.

Occurrence - Isolated from apparently normal rodent fur in Venezuela and from soil in Romania, probably world-wide.

Critical Characteristics - (1) Cashew-nut shaped microaleuriospores, (2) Pycnidia.

References:

Borelli, D. and Frey, M., 1966. Trichophyton phaseoliforme, nova. Species. Medicina Cutanea 2:165-172.

Alteras, I. and Evolceanu, R., 1969. Trichophyton phaseoliforme (Dante, Borelli and Feo, 1966) in Romanian Soil. Mykosen 12:421-426.

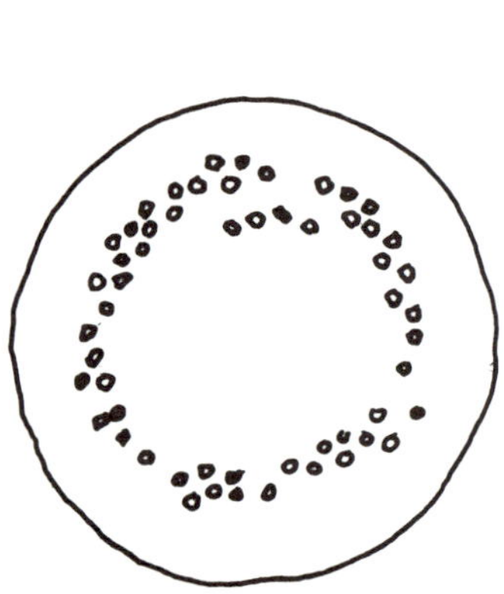

thallus with "pycnidia"

Identification of Trichophyton proliferans

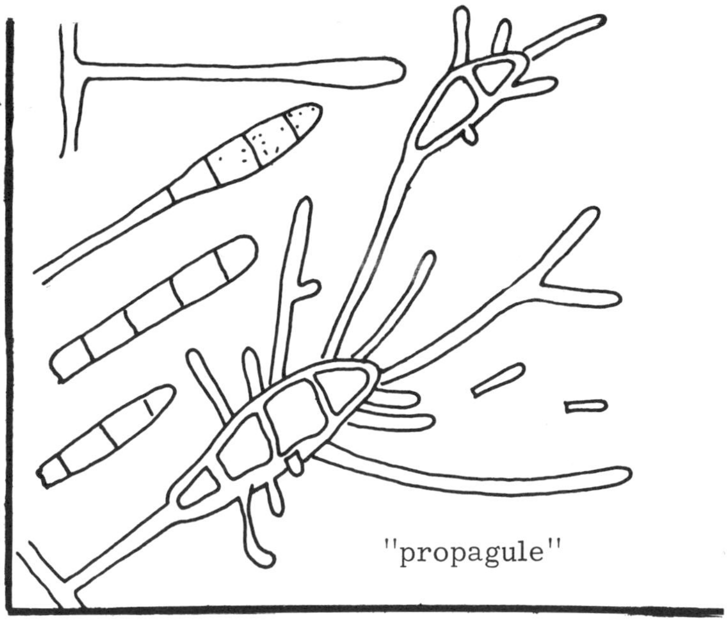

Appearance of Thallus - The white, fluffy, thallus develops surface folds and a slightly faint lemon yellow or buff tint. The undersurface of the thallus, like some other geophilic species such as (A. cuniculi, T. terrestre, etc.), and like T. erinacei, may develop a clear greenish-yellow diffusing pigment, usually becomes deep chrome-yellow as the thallus matures.

Microscopic Morphology - The macroaleuriospores are characteristically small and tapered toward their attachment to the hyphae, with the tip frequently somewhat spindle-shaped and appearing slightly roughened. When detached, the macroaleuriospores range from small one-celled rods, through various short spindle-shaped fusiform structures, to well-developed cylindrical macroaleuriospores of the Trichophyton type. Although single celled clavate elements are present, clearly differentiated microaleuriospores are not found. The most distinctive feature of T. phaseoliforme is the presence of "propagules", which are lateral, multicelled, cylindrical, or spindle-shaped structures in the depths of the thallus. These give rise to multiple frond-like hyphae. The propagules suggest in appearance the perforating organs associated with the saprophytic invasion of the hair by other dermatophytes.

Occurrence - Two children infected in England and one in New Zealand. (Personal communication from F. M. Rush-Munro). The lesions were on the knees, which suggests that T. proliferans may be present in soil.

Critical Characteristics - (1) Propagules, (2) Macroaleuriospores.

Reference:

England, M. P. and Stockdale, P. M., 1968. Trichophyton proliferans sp. nov. A Human Pathogen, Sabouraudia 6:267-270.

Identification of Trichophyton longifusus

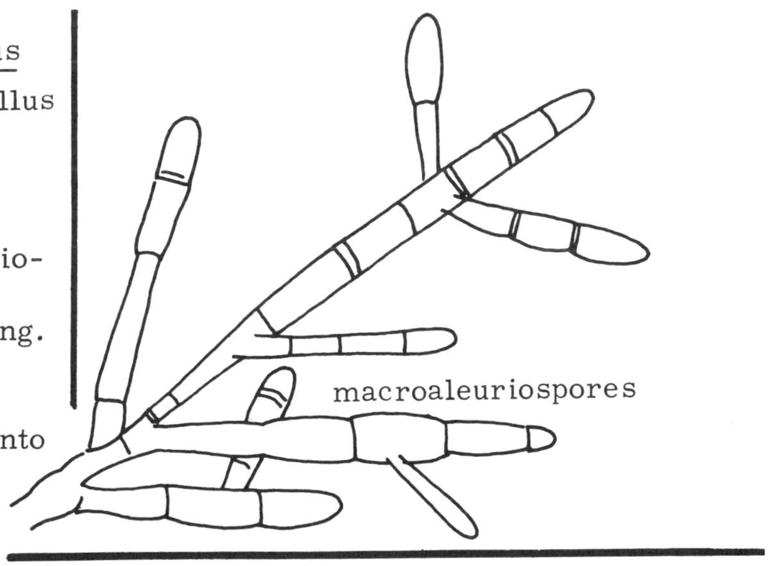

Appearance of Thallus - Surface of thallus fluffy to powdery, and white to pale yellowish, undersurface yellowish brown.

Microscopic Morphology - Macroaleuriospores distinctive, long cylindrical 7 - 9μ in diameter and up to 300μ long. The macroaleuriospores occur in clusters and characteristically may arise from one another and merge into the terminal hyphae suggestive of some isolates of T. rubrum. No microaleuriospores seen.

Trichophyton longifusus - Cont.

Occurrence - Isolated three times in Hungary, twice from soil and once from tinea capitis in presence of M. gypseum.

Comment - The thin-walled macroaleuriospores separate T. longifusus from T. ajelloi.

Critical Characteristics - (1) Macroaleuriospores, (2) Appearance of thallus.

Reference:

Florian, E. and Galgoczy, J., 1964 - 65. Keratinomyces longifusus sp. nov. from Hungary. Mycopath. et Mycologia Applicata 24:73-80.

Identification of Trichophyton thuringiense

Appearance of Thallus - A brownish-red powdery thallus.

Microscopic Morphology - This is a T. terrestre-like species, with large lateral club-shaped microaleuriospores, which show various transitional forms with longer multiseptate macroaleuriospores.

Occurrence - Isolated from normal hair of mice in Europe.

Comment - T. thuringiense does not produce ascospores with tester strains of either A. quadifidum or A. lenticularum, and is otherwise distinguished by the reddish-brown thallus.

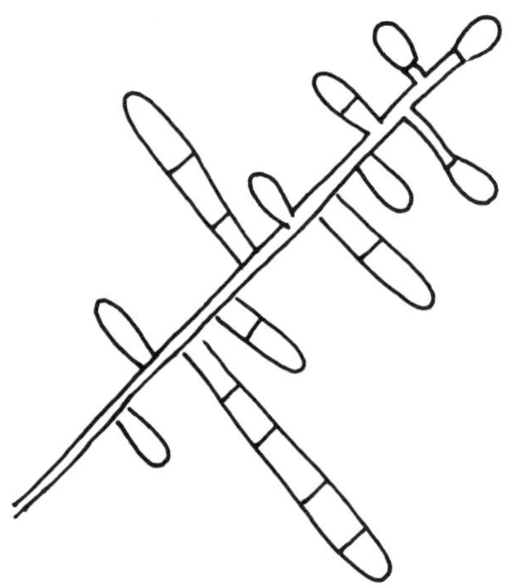

micro- and macroaleuriospores

Critical Characteristics - (1) Microscopic morphology, (2) Appearance of thallus, (3) Failure to produce ascospores with known species of Arthroderma in the T. terrestre complex.

Reference:

Koch, H.A., 1969. Trichophyton thuringiense Spec. nov. Mykosen 12:287-290.

Identification of Trichophyton fluviomuniense

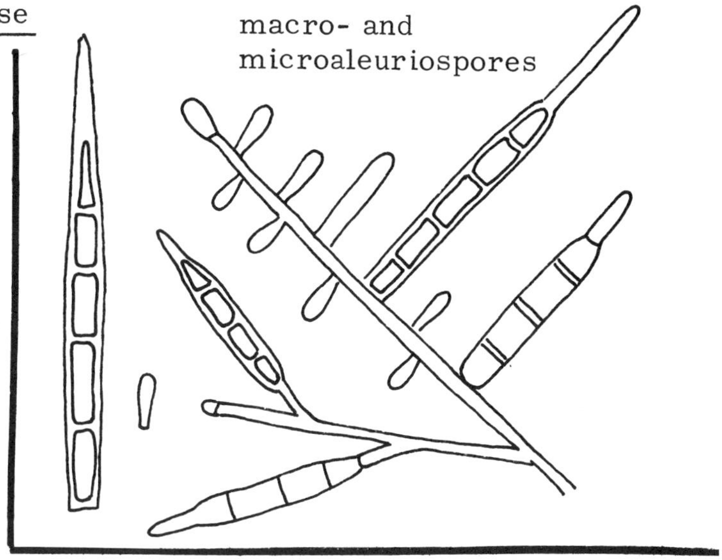

Appearance of Thallus - A reddish-brown thallus with a granular surface, which develops folds and fine cracks centrally with maturity.

Microscopic Morphology - This species is suggestive of T. terrestre, T. tonsurans, and T. megninii. The egg-shaped to club-shaped microaleuriospores show T. terrestre-like transitional forms to multiseptate macroaleuriospores. However, the well-formed macroaleuriospores are long cylindrical structures, frequently tapered or developing a filament at the tip as in some strains of T. mentagrophytes. Development of macroaleuriospores may be favored by 26°C and that of microaleuriospores favored by 37°C.

Occurrence - Isolated from ringworm lesion of a patient from Rio Muni on the west coast of Africa.

Comment - This isolate has been carefully studied and compared with other dermatophytes and appears to be distinct from both T. megninii and T. tonsurans to which it bears perhaps the closest similarity. It does not require histidine or thiamine.

Critical Characteristics - (1) Microscopic morphology, (2) Appearance of thallus, (3) Autotrophy.

Reference:

Miguens, M. P., 1968. Un Neuvo Dermatofite de Origin Tropical; Trichophyton fluviomuniense sp. nov. Sabouraudia 6:312-317.

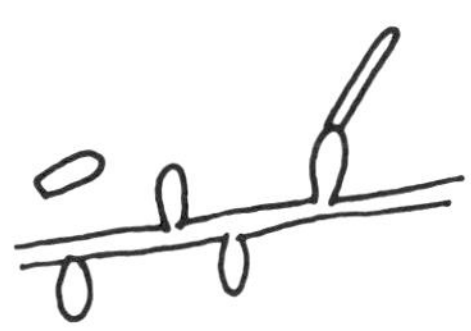

microaleuriospore
with filament

ADDITIONAL SPECIES OF ARTHRODERMA

Differential description of Arthroderma species without named Trichophyton conidial states and Ctenomyces serratus, a related fungus.

I. With well-differentiated large (11 X 50μ±) macroaleuriospores of the Trichophyton type produced terminally on hyphal branches, but no microaleuriospores. Thallus flat with circular growth rings, white to yellow-buff beneath. From feathers of Australian birds. Heterothallic. Peridial hyphae with asymmetric, dumbbell-shaped cells. . . . . Arthroderma flavescens

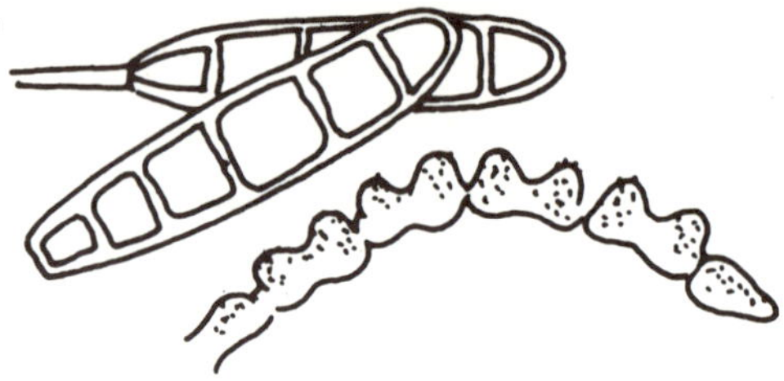

II. With T. terrestre-type morphology. Small, lateral, two to three celled lateral macroaleuriospores, poorly differentiated from abundant clavate, truncate-based microaleuriospores. Thallus flat, densely powdery, white to cream. Keratinophilic, from the environs of birds and mammals. Heterothallic. Peridial hyphae with asymmetric, dumbbell-shaped cells. (See also T. terrestre). . . . . Arthroderma cuniculi

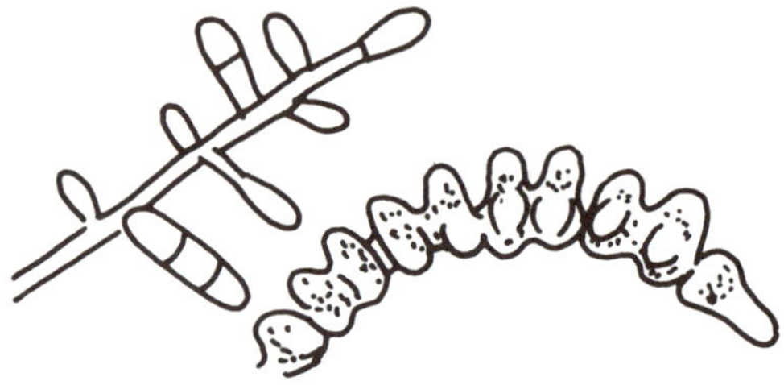

III. Aleuriospores of the Chrysosporium type, large, obovoid, walls smooth, single to triple celled, terminal, lateral and intercalary. Thallus flat, sparsely powdery, white to yellow. Keratinophilic, from the environs of birds and mammals. Heterothallic. Peridial hyphae with asymmetric, dumbbell-shaped cells with multiple tubercles. . . Arthroderma multifidum

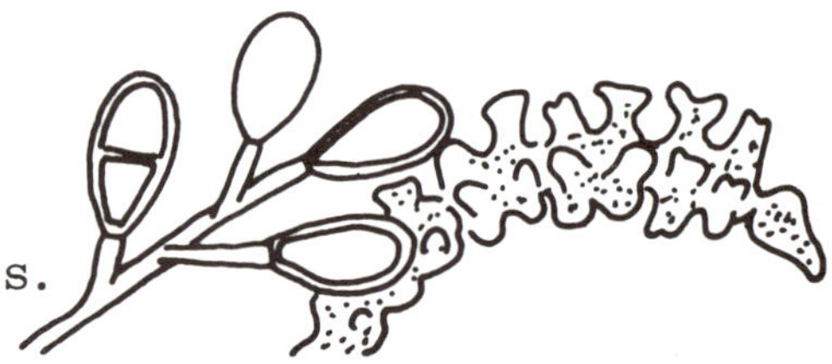

IV. Aleuriospores of the Chrysosporium type, large, walls rough or tuberculate, obovoid to spherical, mainly single-celled. Thallus flat, powdery, white to lemon yellow. Keratinophilic, in soil. Peridial hyphae with asymmetric dumbbell-shaped cells. . . . . Arthroderma tuberculatum

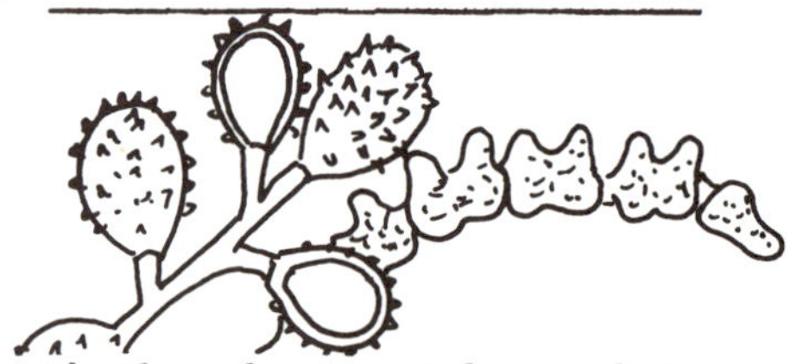

V. Aleuriospores of the Chrysosporium type, large, rough-walled, obovoid, terminal, lateral, and intercallary. Thallus flat, powdery, white to cream colored. Keratinophilic, from the environs of birds and mammals. Homothallic. Peridial hyphae with asymmetric dumbbell-shaped cells and tending to assume a spiral form, and with comb-like appendages. . . . . . . Arthroderma curreyi

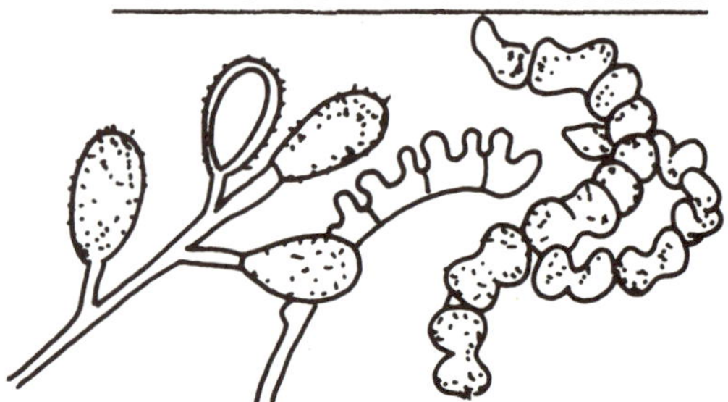

VI. Aleuriospores of the Chrysosporium type, large, rough-walled, obovoid to spherical, terminal, lateral, and intercallary. Thallus usually slow growing and buff to olive-buff in color. Keratinophilic, soil and feathers. Heterothallic. Peridial hyphae with long, comb-like projections. A fungus once confused with A. curreyi and with the perfect state of dermatophytes. . . . . Ctenomyces serratus

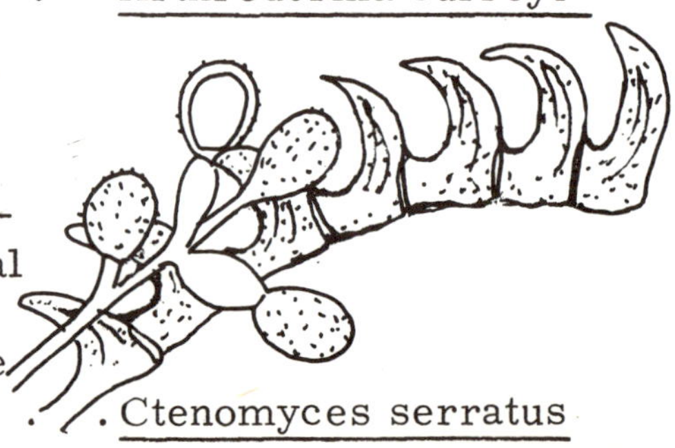

KERATINOPHILIC SPECIES OF CHRYSOSPORIUM

The genus Chrysosporium has been less studied than the dermatophytes, so that a list of species cannot be compiled with the same confidence. The standard reference is Carmichael, J. W., 1962, Canadian J. Botany 40: 1137-1172. In this manual we have limited ourselves to a discussion of keratinophilic species, which includes all the known Arthroderma species with unnamed Chrysosporium states (see opposite page). These fungi and some of the arthroaleuriospore-producing fungi discussed on page 73 may resemble T. mentagrophytes macroscopically and are obtained as contaminants in cultures from skin lesions. They usually have the properties of the dermatophytes listed on page 5.

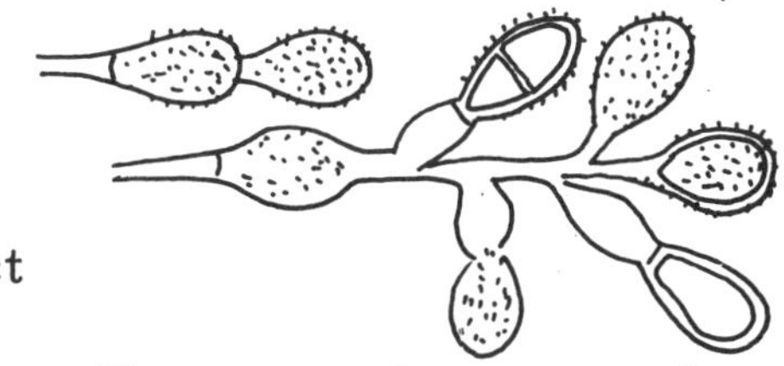

I. Aleuriospores large, egg-shaped, rough or echinulate, frequently with swollen stalks, resembling those of Ctenomyces serratus. Perfect state unknown. Digests hair without forming perforating organs. . . . . Chrysosporium asperatum

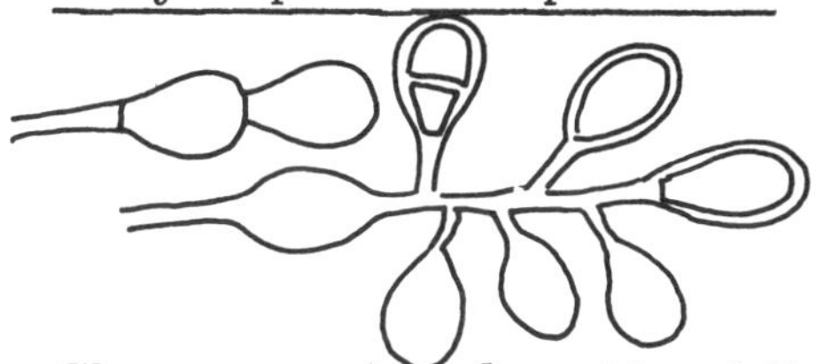

II. Aleuriospores large, egg-shaped, mostly smooth resembling those of Arthroderma multifidum. Thallus flat, powdery, white to cream. Digests hair, but does not produce perforating organs. Poor growth at 37°C. . . . . Chrysosporium keratinophilum

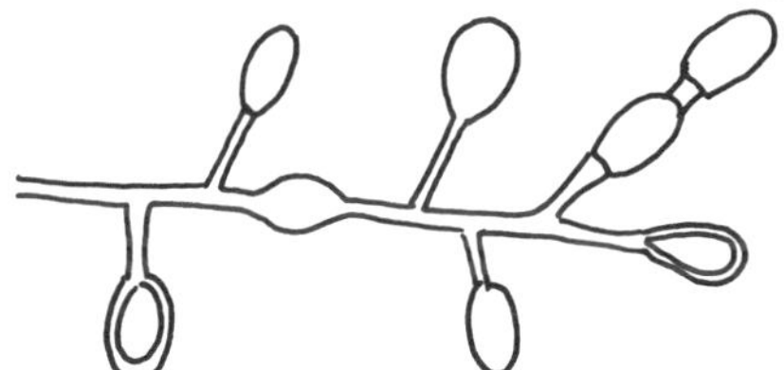

III. Aleuriospores small, smooth, or somewhat variable in size, suggesting a small size edition of C. keratinophilum. Thallus flat, powdery, white to cream. Perfect state unknown. Good growth at 37°C. . . . . Chrysosporium tropicum

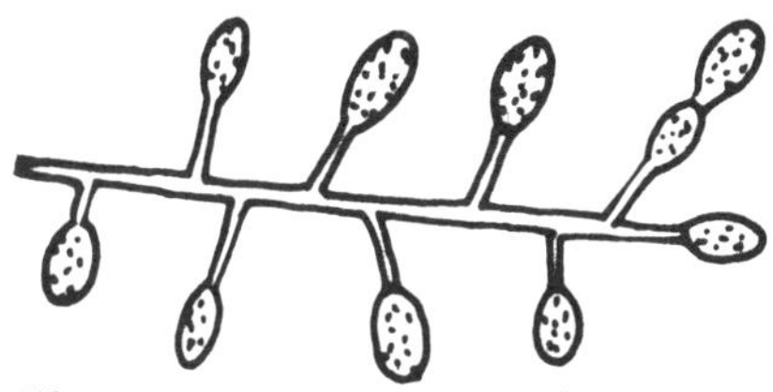

IV. Aleuriospores approaching in size those of C. tropicum, but rough or finely echinulate and tending to be oat shaped and pointed, rather than egg-shaped, suggesting a large size edition of C. indicum. Thallus flat, powdery, white to cream. Perfect state unknown. . . . . . Chrysosporium evolceanui

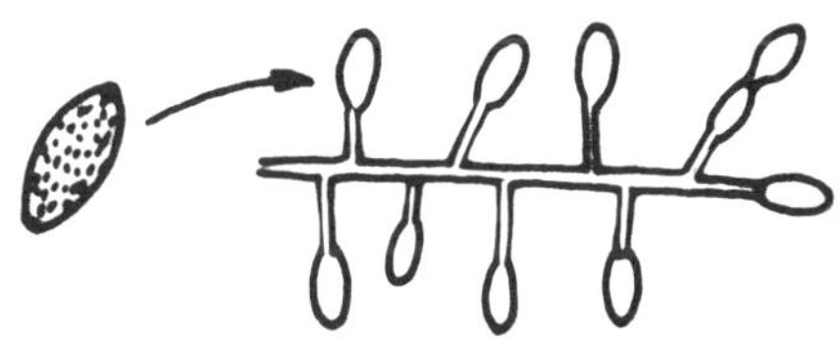

V. Aleuriospores small, finely echinulate, and mostly oat-shaped. Thallus flat, powdery, white to cream. Perfect state Aphanoascus terreus, homothallic? Ascocarp places fungus in the Cephalothecaceae rather than in the Gymnoascaceae. Plate IV. . . . . Chrysosporium indicum

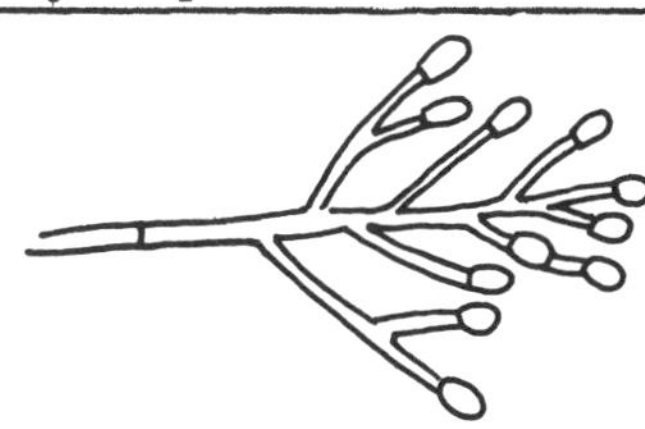

VI. Aleuriospores rounded, club-shaped, smooth or roughened, and produced in terminal clusters or panicles with branches forward directed. Perfect state uncertain. Isolated by hair bait technique from soil and as laboratory contaminant. Does not digest hair or grow at 37°C. Digests cellulose. Chrysosporium pannorum

Keratinophilic Species - Cont.

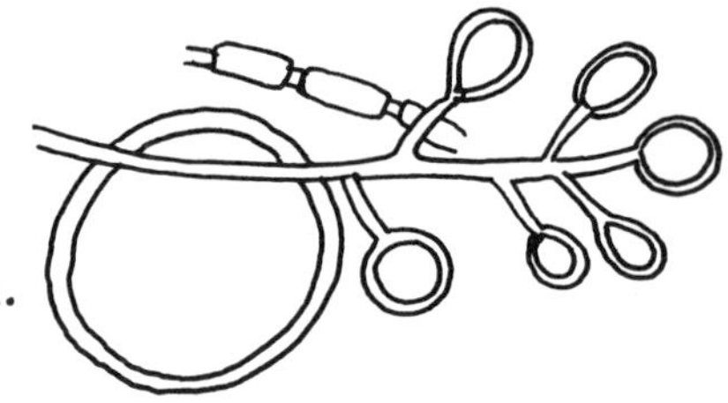

VII. Aleuriospores rounded to spherical, variable in size from strain to strain. Arthroaleuriospores frequently abundant. Thallus flat powdery, white to cream. Perfect state unknown. Grows well at 37 - 45°C, frequently with formation of large spherical chlamydospores. Digests cellulose rather than hair. . . . . . Chrysosporium pruinosum

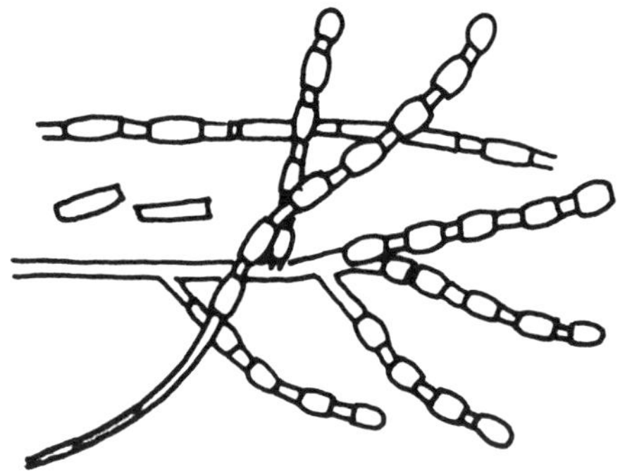

Malbranchea spp.

VIII. Arthroaleuriospores are frequent in some dermatophyte cultures, especially T. rubrum, M. canis, T. mentagrophytes, and T. gloriae. Unless micro- and macroaleuriospores are seen such cultures resemble the geophilic fungus Malbranchea, in which branched terminal chains of arthroaleuriospores (alternate arthrospores) are the principal type of spore. Catenulate aleuriospores are formed in most cultures of Chrysosporium. Up to date taxonomic information about both Chrysosporium and Malbranchea should be obtained from current literature rather than from this manual, which merely provides an introduction to the better known species as they relate to dermatophytes and their identification. Publications on Arthroderma, Chrysosporium, etc. are included among the references which follow. In general fungi in the family Gymnoascaceae (many of which have Chrysosporium and arthroaleuriospore conidial states) are frequently obtained from the soil by the hair bait technique and constitute taxonomic relatives of the dermatophytes.

REFERENCES TO ORIGINAL TAXONOMIC DESCRIPTIONS

Aphanoascus terreus (Randhawa and Sandu, 1964) Apinis, 1968: Sabouraudia , 3, 251-256 and Mycopath. Mycol. Appl., 35, 97-104.

Arthroderma benhamiae Ajello & Cheng, 1967: See page 42.
A. ciferrii Varsavsky & Ajello, 1964: See page 35.

A. cuniculi Dawson, 1963: Sabouraudia, 2, 185-191.

A. curreyi Berkeley, 1860: "Outlines of British Fungology", page 357, Lovell Reeve, London; (see also Dawson, C.O. & Gentles, J.C., 1961: Sabouraudia, 1, 49-57 and Stockdale, P.M., 1961: Sabouraudia, 1, 41-48).

A. flavescens Rees, 1967: Sabouraudia, 5, 206-208.

A. gertleri Bohme, 1967: See page 37.
A. gloriae Ajello, 1967: See page 36.

A. lenticularum Pore, Tsao & Plunkett, 1965: See page 34.

A. multifidum Dawson, 1963: Sabouraudia, 2, 185-191.

A. quadrifidum Dawson & Gentles, 1961: See page 34.
A. simii Stockdale, Mackenzie & Austwick, 1965: See page 39.

A. tuberculatum Kuehn, 1960: Mycopathologia, 13, 189-197.

A. uncinatum Dawson & Gentles, 1961: See page 32.

Chrysosporium asperatum Carmichael, 1962: Canad. J. Bot., 40, 1137-1173.

C. evolceanui (Randhawa & Sandhu, 1963) Garg, 1960: Mycopath. Mycol. Appl. 20, 225-238; and Sabouraudia 4, 259-264. (See also Zeller, L., 1968: Mycopath. Mycol. Appl. 34:296-301).

C. indicum (Randhawa & Sandhu, 1963) Garg, 1966: Mycopath. Mycol. Appl. 20, 225-238; and Sabouraudia 4, 259-264.

C. keratinophilum (Frey, 1961) Carmichael, 1962: Mycologia, 51, 641; and Canad. J. Bot., 40, 1137-1173.

C. pannorum (Link, 1824) Hughes, 1958: Linn spec. Plant. IV 6, 1-73; and Canad. J. Botany, 36, 749-836.

C. pruinosom (Gilman and Abott, 1927) Carmichael, 1962. Iowa State Coll. J. Sci., 1, 306; and Canad. J. Botany, 40, 1137-1173.

C. tropicum, Carmichael, 1962: Canad. J. Bot., 40, 1137-1173.

Ctenomyces serratus, Eidan, 1880: Frey and Griffin, 1961. Trans. Brit. Mycol. Soc., 44, 449-452 and Orr and Kuehn 1963. Mycopath. Mycol. Appl. 21, 321-333.

Epidermophyton floccosum (Harz, 1870) Langeron & Milochevitch, 1930: Bull Soc. Imp. Nat. Moscou, 44, 88-147; and Ann. Parasit.hum.comp., 8, 465-508.

Malbranchea spp. (Saccardo, 1882) (See Cooney, D. G. and Emerson, R. "Thermophilic Fungi", W. H. Freeman and Co., San Francisco, 188 pp., 1964; and Wang, C. J. K., "Fungi of Pulp and Paper in New York", State University College of Forestry at Syracuse University Technical Publication No. 87, 1965.

Microsporum amazonicum Moraes, Borelli & Feo, 1967: See page 65.

M. audouinii Gruby, 1843: C.R. Acad. Sci., Paris, 17, 301-303.

M. boullardii Dominik & Majchrowicz, 1965: See page 63.

M. canis Bodin, 1902: "Les champignons parasites de l'homme". Masson et Cie, Paris.

M. cookei Ajello, 1959: See page 29.

M. distortum Di Menna & Marples, 1954: Trans. Br. mycol. Soc., 37, 372-374.

M. ferrugineum Ota, 1921: Zap. Zeit, Derm., Urol, 21, 201, 330, 340.

M. fulvum Uriburu 1909: Argent. Med., Buenos Aires, 7, 563-582.

M. gypseum (Bodin, 1907) Guiart & Grigorakis, 1928: Ann. Derm. Syph, 8, 585-602; and Lyon med., 141, 369-378.

M. nanum Fuentes, 1956: Mycologia, 48, 613-614.

M. persicolor (Sabouraud, 1910) Guiart & Grigorakis, 1928: "Les Teignes". Masson et Cie, Paris; and Lyon Med., 141, 369-378.

M. praecox Rivalier, 1954: See page 64.

M. racemosum Borelli, 1965: See page 55.

M. vanbreuseghemii Georg, Ajello, Freidman & Brinkman, 1962: See page 30.

Nannizzia cajetani Ajello, 1961: See page 29.

N. fulva Stockdale, 1963: See page 25.

N. grubyia Georg, Ajello & Brinkman, 1962: See page 30.

N. incurvata Stockdale, 1961: See page 24.

N. gypsea Stockdale, 1963: See page 24.

N. obtusa Dawson & Gentles, 1961: See page 26.

N. persicolor Stockdale, 1967: See page 28.

References - Cont.

Trichophyton ajelloi (Vanbreuseghem, 1952) Ajello, 1968: Bull Acad. roy. Med. Belg., 38, 1068-1077; and Sabouraudia, 6, 147-159.

T. concentricum Blanchard, 1895: Traité de pathologie générale, 2, 811-926, Masson et Cie, Paris.

T. equinum (Matruchot & Dassonville, 1898) Gedoelst, 1902: C.R. Acad. Sci. Paris, 127, 279-281; and "Les champignons parasites de l'homme et des animaux domestiques". Joseph Van In & Cie, Lierre.

T. fluviomuniense Miguens, 1968: See page 69.

T. gallinae (Megnin, 1881) Silva & Benham, 1952: C.R. Soc. Biol, Paris, 33, 404-406; and J. Invest. Derm., 18, 453-472.

T. georgiae Varsavsky & Ajello, 1964: See page 35.
T. gloriae Ajello and Cheng, 1967: See page 36.
T. gourvilii Catanei, 1933: See page 55.

T. longifusus (Florian & Galgoczy, 1964) Ajello, 1968: See page 68; and Sabouraudia, 6, 147-159.

T. megninii Blanchard, 1896: Traité de pathologie générale, 2, 811-926, Masson et Cie, Paris.

T. mentagrophytes (Robin, 1853) Blanchard, 1896: "Histoire naturelle des vegétaux parastites qui croissent sur l'homme et sur les animaux vivants". J. B. Baillière, Paris; and Traite de pathologie générale, 2, 811-926, Masson et Cie, Paris.

T. phaseoliforme Borelli & Feo, 1966: See page 66.
T. proliferans English & Stockdale, 1968: See page 67.

T. rubrum (Castellani, 1910) Sabouraud, 1911: J. Derm. Syph., 22, 147-150; and Br. J. Derm., 23, 389-390.

T. schoenleinii (Lebert, 1845) Langeron & Milochevitch, 1930: "Memorie sur la teigne", 2, 477-497; and Ann. Parasit. hum. comp., 8, 465-508.

T. simii (Pinoy, 1912) Stockdale, Mackenzie & Austwick, 1965: C.R. Soc. Biol. Paris, 72, 59; and see page 39.

T. soudanense Joyeux, 1912: C.R. Soc. Biol. Paris, 73, 15-16.

T. terrestre Durie & Frey, 1957: See page 34.
T. thuringiense Koch, 1969: See page 68.

T. tonsurans Malmsten, 1845: Arch. Anat. Physiol. Wiss. Med., 1848, 1-19.

T. vanbreuseghemii Rioux, Jarry & Juminer, 1964: See page 37.

T. verrucosum Bodin, 1902: "Les champignons parasites de l'homme". Masson et Cie, Paris.

T. violaceum Bodin, 1902: "Les champignons parasites de l'homme". Masson et Cie, Paris.

T. yaoundei Cochet & Doby-Dubois, 1957: Sem.Hôp. Paris, 33, 26-30.

PLATE ONE

Microsporum species

13

Microsporum
canis
Sabouraud's
Agar
with yeast
extract

15

Microsporum
distortum
Sabouraud's
Agar
with yeast
extract

16

Microsporum
audouinii
Sabouraud's
Agar

16

Microsporum
audouinii
var. rivalierii
Cycloheximide
Agar (Mycosel)

19

Microsporum
ferrugineum
(Asiatic type)
Sabouraud's
Agar
with yeast
extract

23

Microsporum
gypseum
(Nannizzia
incurvata)
Sabouraud's
Agar

23

Microsporum
gypseum
(Nannizzia
gypsea)
Sabouraud's
Agar

25

Microsporum
fulvum
Sabouraud's
Agar
with yeast
extract

26

Microsporum
nanum
Sabouraud's
Agar
with yeast
extract

29

Microsporum
cookei
Sabouraud's
Agar
with yeast
extract

30

Microsporum
van-
breuseghemii
Sabouraud's
Agar

16

Microsporum
audouinii
var. langeronii
Sabouraud's
Agar
with yeast
extract

Photographed by Vivienne Roberts
Department of Medical Illustration
University of Miami School of Medicine

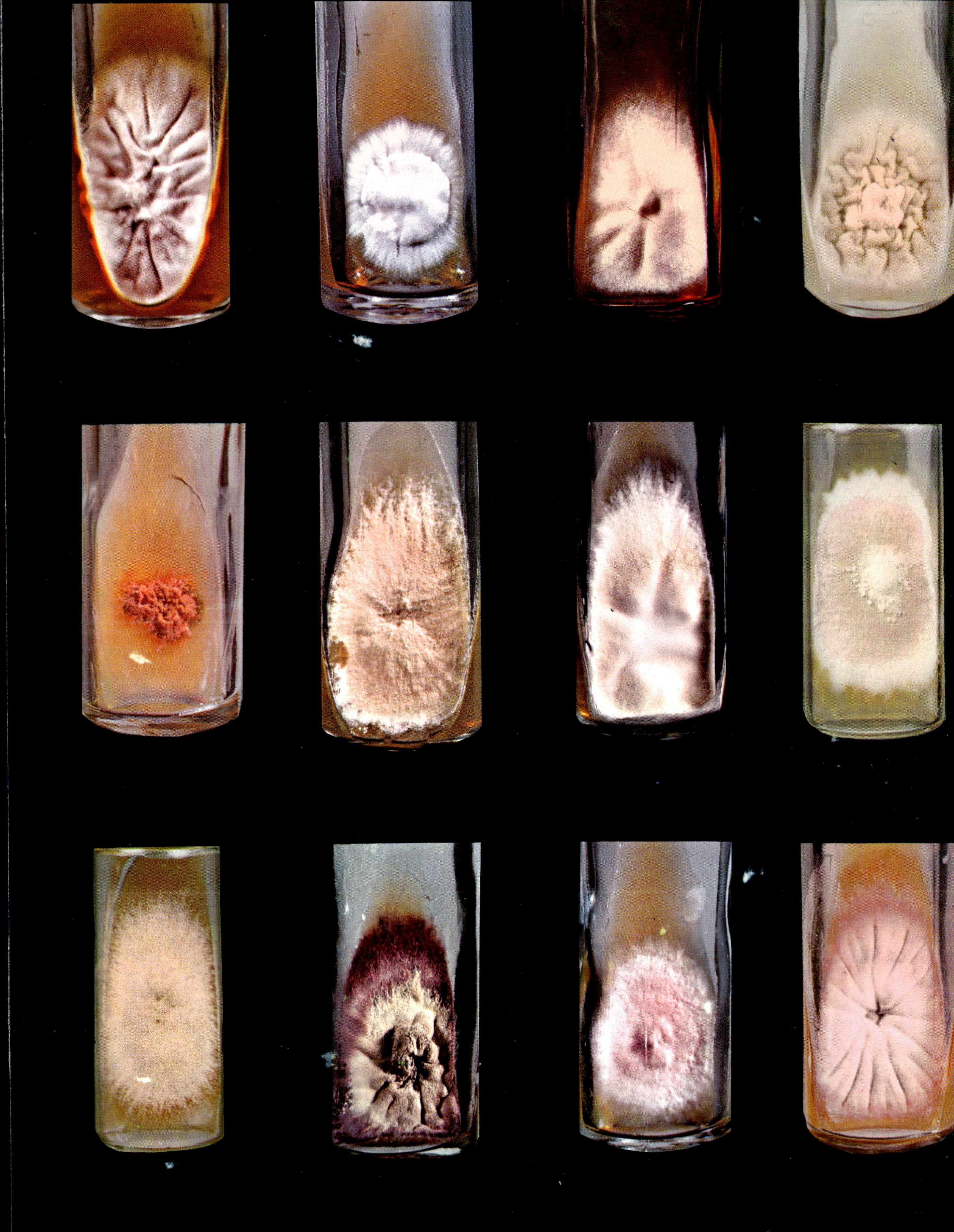

PLATE TWO

Trichophyton terrestre, ectothrix Trichophyton species

and Trichophyton (Microsporum?) gallinae

33 Trichophyton terrestre (hedgehog form) Sabouraud's Agar with yeast extract	33 Trichophyton terrestre Sabouraud's Agar with yeast extract	40 Trichophyton menta- grophytes zoophilic form Sabouraud's Agar	40 Trichophyton menta- grophytes tinea pedis form Sabouraud's Agar
44 Trichophyton erinacei Sabouraud's Agar with yeast extract (surface of colony)	44 Trichophyton erinacei Sabouraud's Agar with yeast extract (back of colony)	45 Trichophyton equinum Sabouraud's Agar with yeast extract (surface of colony)	45 Trichophyton equinum Sabouraud's Agar with yeast extract (back of colony)
47 Trichophyton verrucosum (album form) Sabouraud's Agar with yeast extract typically more chalky	47 Trichophyton verrucosum (ochraceum form) Sabouraud's Agar with yeast extract	21 Trichophyton (M?) gallinae Sabouraud's Agar	49 Trichophyton megninii Sabouraud's Agar

Photographed by Vivienne Roberts
Department of Medical Illustration
University of Miami School of Medicine

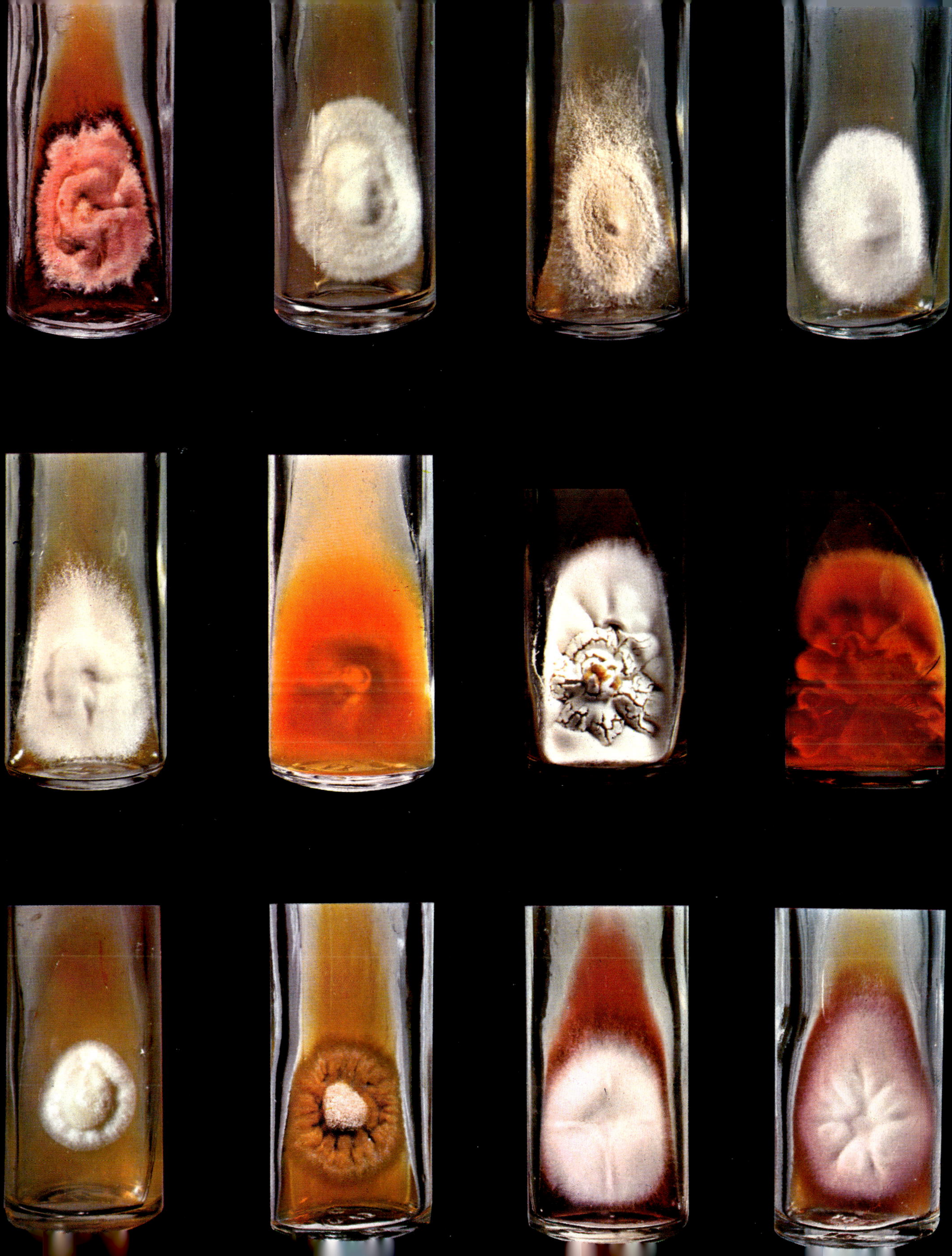

PLATE THREE

Trichophyton rubrum, endothrix Trichophyton species, Trichophyton schoenleinii, Trichophyton concentricum and Epidermophyton floccosum

50

Trichophyton rubrum (fluffy form) Sabouraud's Agar

50

Trichophyton rubrum (granular form) Sabouraud's Agar with yeast extract

52

Trichophyton tonsurans Sabouraud's Agar with yeast extract

52

Trichophyton tonsurans (sulfureum form) Sabouraud's Agar with yeast extract

54

Trichophyton violaceum Sabouraud's Agar with yeast extract

55

Trichophyton gourvilii Sabouraud's Agar

56

Trichophyton soudanense Sabouraud's Agar with yeast extract

58

Trichophyton yaoundei Sabouraud's Agar with yeast extract

typically more glabrous

59

Trichophyton schoenleinii Sabouraud's Agar with yeast extract

initial isolates more convoluted

61

Trichophyton concentricum Sabouraud's Agar with yeast extract

62

Epidermophyton floccosum Sabouraud's Agar with yeast extract

50

Trichophyton rubrum (isolate producing brown pigment) Sabouraud's Agar with yeast extract

Photographed by Vivienne Roberts
Department of Medical Illustration
University of Miami School of Medicine

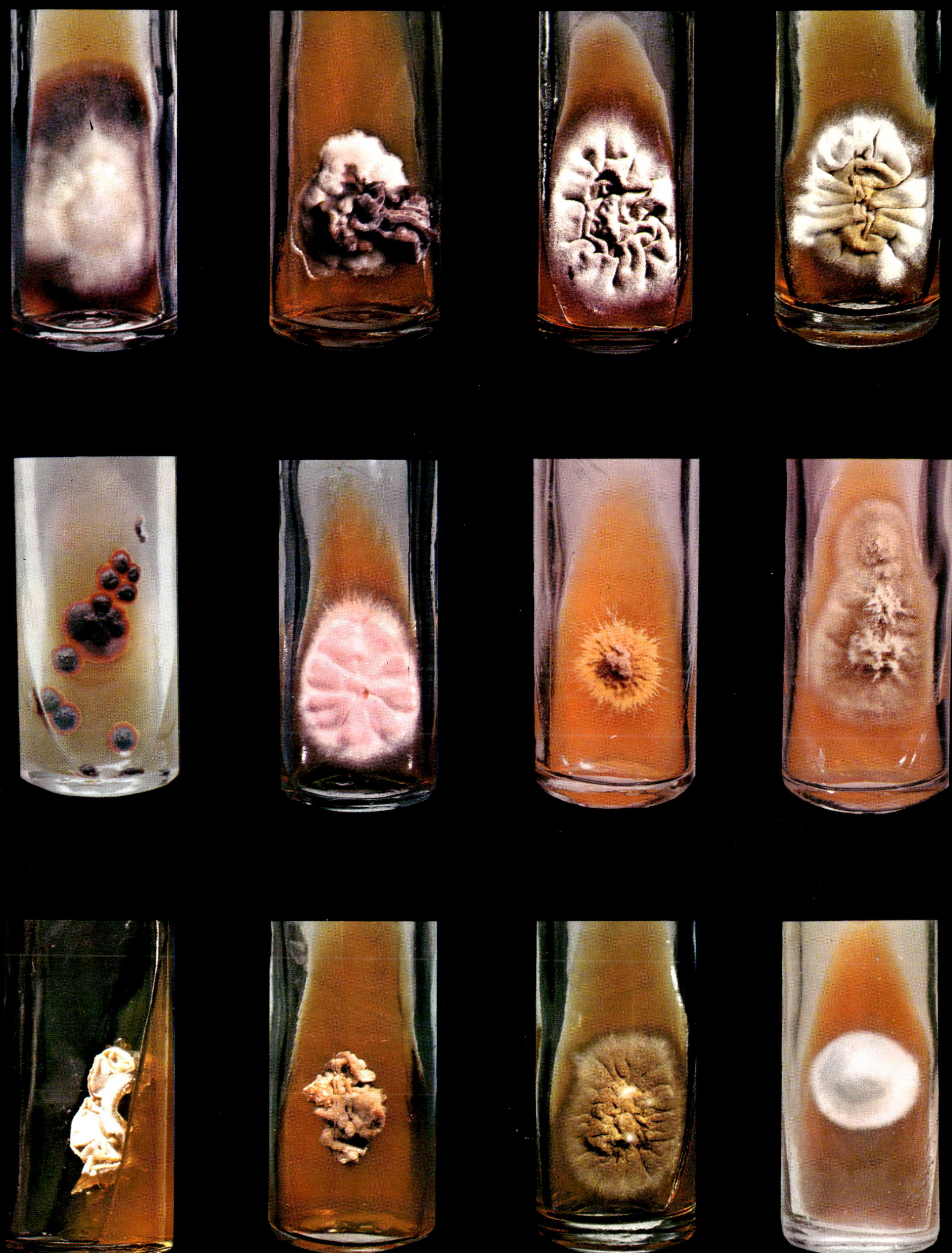

PLATE FOUR

Primary Outgrowths of Common Dermatophytes

Additional Ascigerous Dermatophytes

23 13 16 40 50 50 52 62

Primary outgrowths on chloramphenicol-cyclohexamide agar: 23 M. gypseum, 13 M. canis, 16 M. audouinii, 40 T. mentagrophytes var. interdigitale, 50 T. rubrum (fluffy types), 52 T. tonsurans (mahogany brown form), 62 E. floccosum.

71 Chrysosporium indicum Sabouraud's Agar with yeast extract

40 Trichophyton mentagrophytes var. nodular Sabouraud's Agar with yeast extract (showing regular fluffy pleomorphic change)

35 Trichophyton georgiae Sabouraud's Agar with yeast extract

64 Microsporum racemosum Sabouraud's Agar with yeast extract

27 Microsporum persicolor Sabouraud's Agar with yeast extract

31 Trichophyton ajelloi Sabouraud's Agar with yeast extract

36 Trichophyton gloriae Sabouraud's Agar with yeast extract

37 Trichophyton vanbreuseghemii Sabouraud's Agar with yeast extract

38 Trichophyton simii Sabouraud's Agar with yeast extract

Photographed by Vivienne Roberts
Department of Medical Illustration
University of Miami School of Medicine

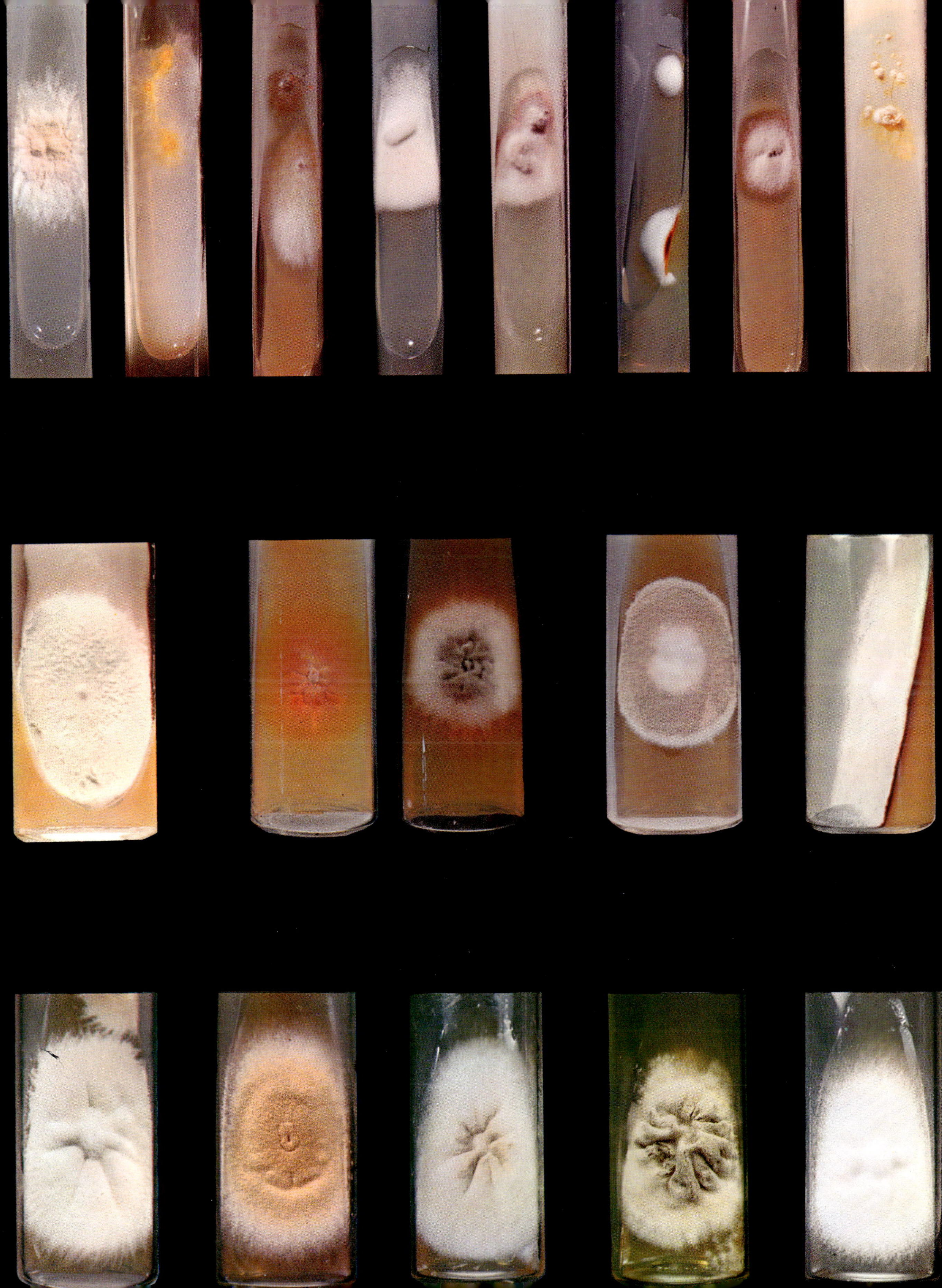

Photomicrographs of Aleuriospores of Dermatophytes

and Related Fungi

Dermatophyte Aleuriospores
(Magnification 700X as printed, 1mm = 1.43μ)

Row A - Thick-Walled Macroaleuriospores
1) M. canis
2) M. distortum - Thick walls not illustrated
3) M. audouinii
4) M. cookei
5) M. vanbreuseghemii
6) T. ajelloi

Row B - Thin-Walled Macroaleuriospores with Rough Walls
7) M. nanum - Note microaleuriospores
8) M. gypseum (broad form)
9) M. persicolor - Note spherical microaleuriospores
10) M. fulvum
11) M. boullardii - Note somewhat thick walls
12) M. racemosum
13) M. amazonicum
14) T. (M?) gallinae - Echinulations not evident on Sabouraud's Agar

Row C -
15) M. gypseum (narrow form)

Row D - Thin-Walled Macroaleuriospores with Smooth Walls
16) E. floccosum
17) T. vanbreuseghemii
18) T. simii
19) T. mentagrophytes
20) T. rubrum (fluffy thallus)
21) E. floccosum

Row E -
22) Chrysosporium indicum - Echinulate surface seen at higher magnification
23) T. gloriae - Macroaleuriospores
24) T. phaseoliforme - Microaleuriospores
25) T. mentagrophytes - Microaleuriospores (immature)
26) T. tonsurans - Microaleuriospores
27) T. rubrum (powdery-suede thallus)

Row F -
28) T. georgiae
29) T. terrestre - Macro- and microaleuriospores
30) Arthroderma tuberculatum (rough) and Chrysosporium keratinophilum (smooth)

Row G -
31) Chrysosporium tropicum
32) T. proliferans - Macroaleuriospores
33) M. persicolor - Microaleuriospores (immature)
34) T. gloriae - Micro- and macroaleuriospores
35) T. rubrum (thallus with macroaleuriospores predominant)

Row H -
36) M. racemosum - Microaleuriospores (immature)

(numbers refer to inked numbers in plate)

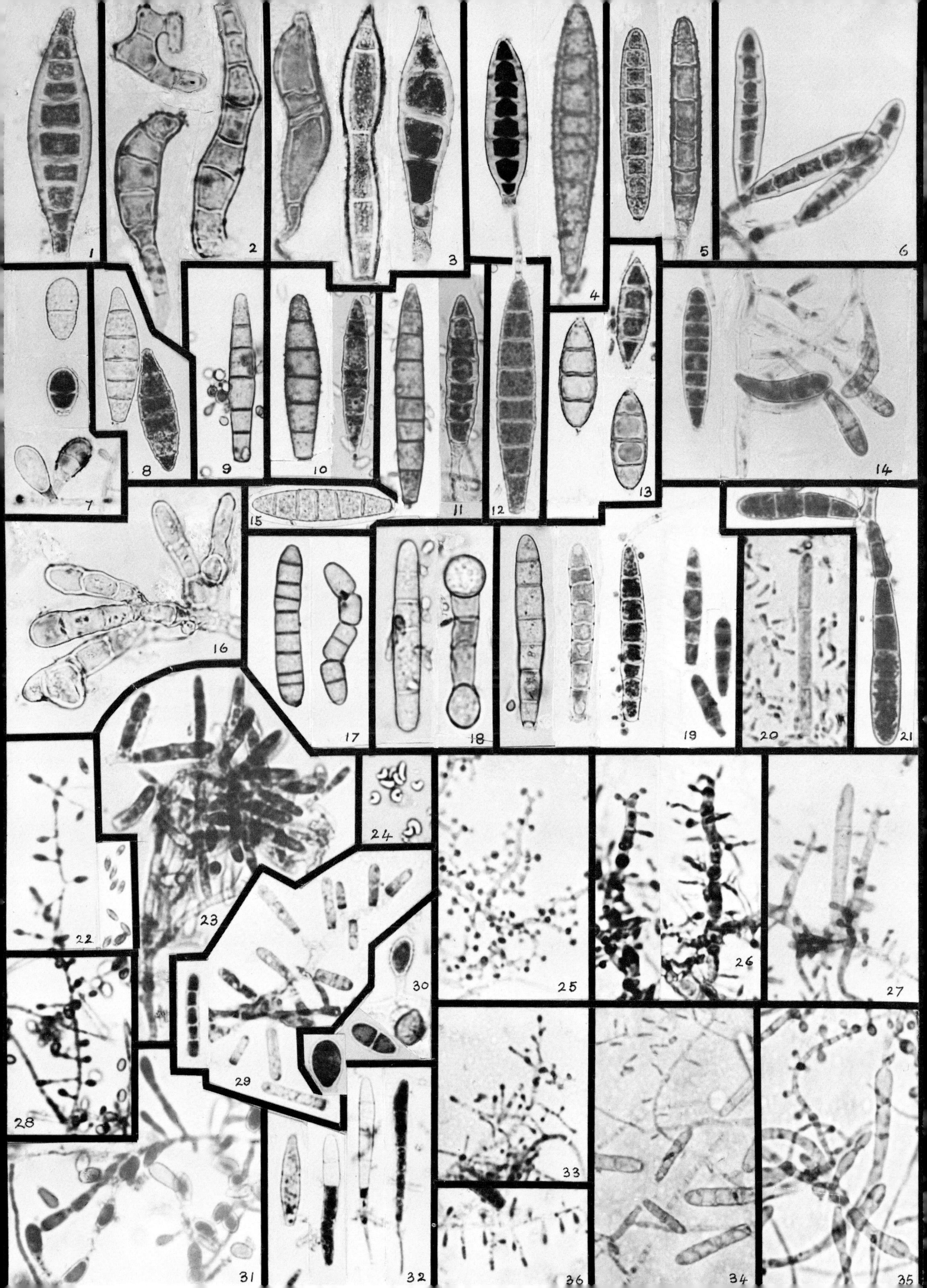
1
2
3
4
5
6
7
8
9
10
11
12
13
14
15
16
17
18
19
20
21
22
23
24
25
26
27
28
29
30
31
32
33
34
35
36

KEY FOR THE IDENTIFICATION OF SPECIES IN THE DERMATOPHYTES, (based on their morphology on Sabouraud's Dextrose Agar incubated at 25 - 30°C)

Introduction

Culture Observation

The most effective use of the key will depend on careful microscopic examination of cultures both in the early stage of growth (or from the active edge of the thallus) and again after the thallus has matured (or from the mature center of a growing thallus). The key may not be applicable to single observations made at any stage of growth.

Numbering

In using the key, follow the **bold face** numbers in the right and left hand margins. These refer to the items in the key. As in other sections of the manual, numbers preceeding species names refer to page numbers in the manual.

Terminology

Terms are defined in the glossary on page 119.

Microscopic Examination

To reveal the cell wall of macroaleuriospores, modified Albert's solution I is recommended, and for examining the normal arrangements of spores on the hyphae a tape mount with lactol phenol cotton blue is usually adequate (methods section, page 114). The photomicrographs on page 81 illustrate some of the distinctions made in the key.

Common Pathogens

The skeleton outline of the key on page 84 may be useful in finding common pathogens. The designations (CHP) anthropophilic or common as human pathogen, (RHP) rare as human pathogen, and (NHP) not recorded as a human pathogen, together with annotations on usual clinical association and geographical distribution, are the only special aids to common clinical isolates in the key itself.

Final Identification

The key is intended mainly as a help to the pages of detailed description most likely to be appropriate to the culture. These descriptions of species should be consulted since they, rather than the key, provide the final guide to identification within the limitations of the manual.

Culture Variants

An attempt has been made to include the common range of variation in the key. Alternatives, designated in the key as "(also check.......)", should be checked, since these attempt to encompass the full range of variation which might be encountered, particularly in parasitic species.

SKELETON OUTLINE OF THE KEY
(THE MORE COMMON HUMAN AND VETERINARY PATHOGENS)

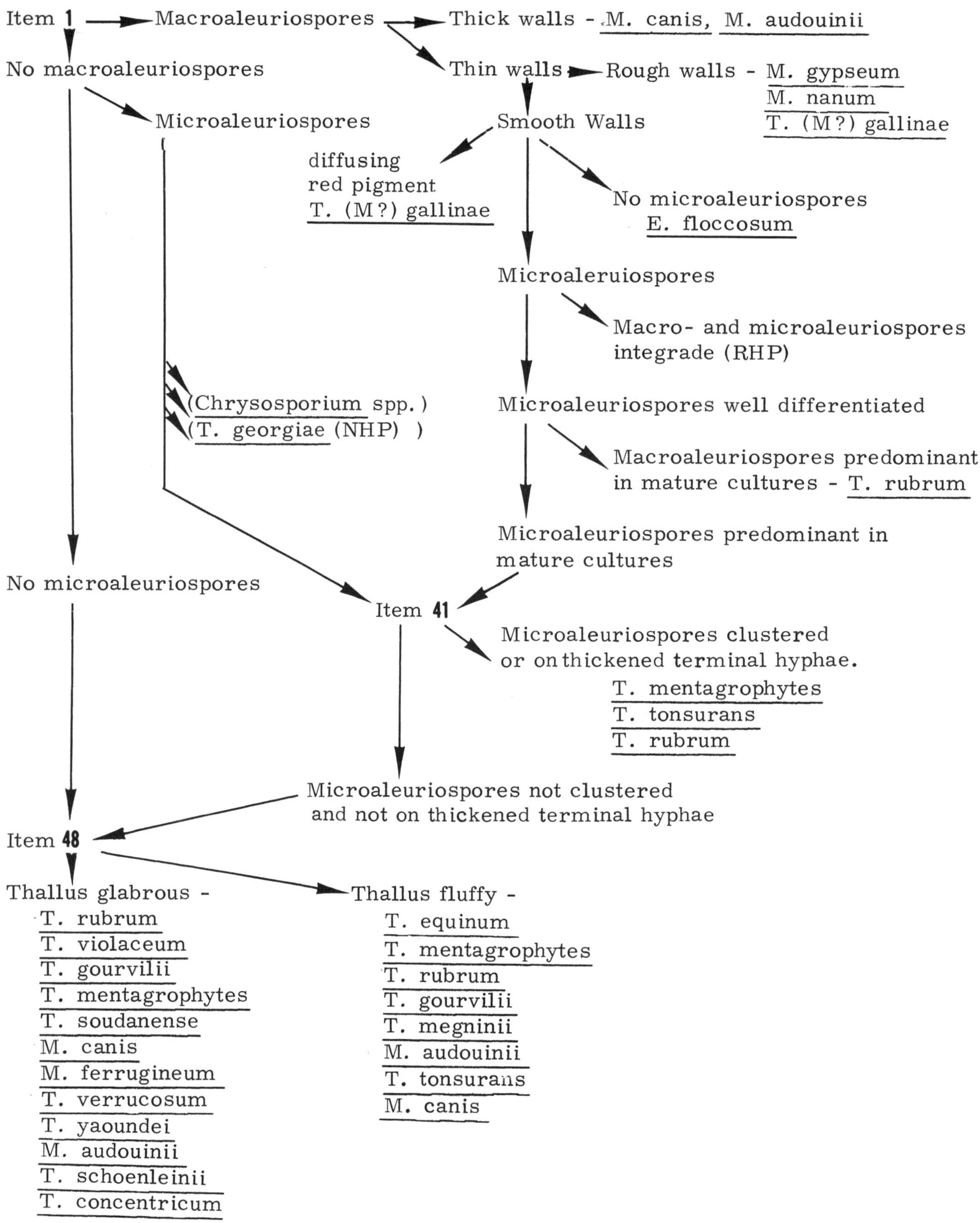

1 Macroaleuriospores (predominantly with 2 or more cells) present 2

Macroaleuriospores absent 34

2 Walls of some or most macroaleuriospores noticibly thicker than the septa (photomicrographs 1 - 6) 3

Walls of macroaleuriospores not thicker than septa (photomicrographs 7 - 21, 23, 27, 29, 32, 34, 35) 10

3 Macroaleuriospores frequently with a distinct beak at tip and spindle-shaped, frequently asymmetric; or else distorted or aborted in shape (photomicrographs 1 - 3). Frequently associated with fluorescent scalp ringworm 4

Macroaleuriospores usually without a terminal beak and symmetrical, spindle-shaped, or long ellipsoidal (photomicrographs 4 - 9) 7

4 Macroaleuriospores spindle-shaped, frequently 75 to 150μ long and with up to 15 cells, usually with terminal beak which is echinulate and often deflected to one side. Microaleuriospores usually not conspicuously abundant. Thallus colorless or more frequently deep yellow beneath (if yellow pigment is absent check 16 M. audouinii). . . 13 M. canis (CHP), cat and other animals (also check 19 M. ferrugineum).

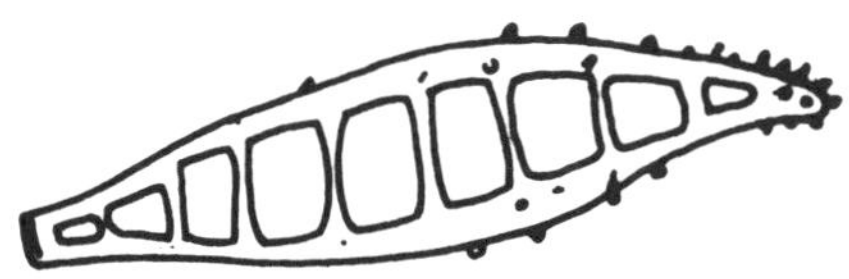

Macroaleuriospores somewhat as above, but aborted, misshapen; or substantially longer than 150μ but with less than 8 cells 5

5 As in M. canis (see item 4), but macroaleuriospores small, blunted (often without terminal beak), aborted, or beaded (frequently with constrictions at the septa). . . 13 M. canis var. obesum (CHP), frequently primates and horses.

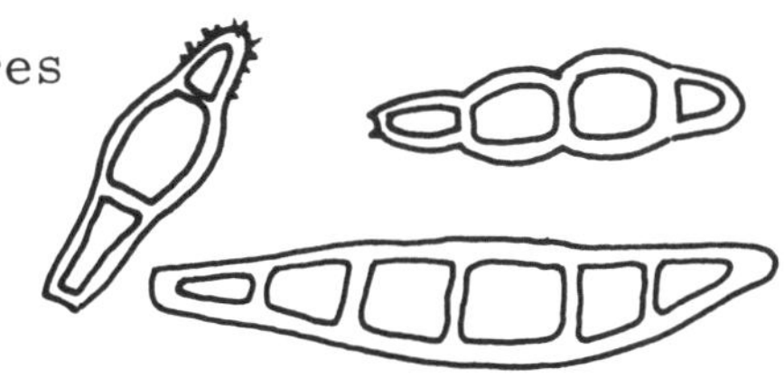

Macroaleuriospores variously misshapen or frequently constricted in midlength (hour-glass or tadpole shape), or longer than 150μ 6

6 Macroaleuriospores variously misshapen. Microaleuriospores sometimes very numerous. Undersurface of thallus white or yellow. . . 15 M. distortum (RHP), man and animals.

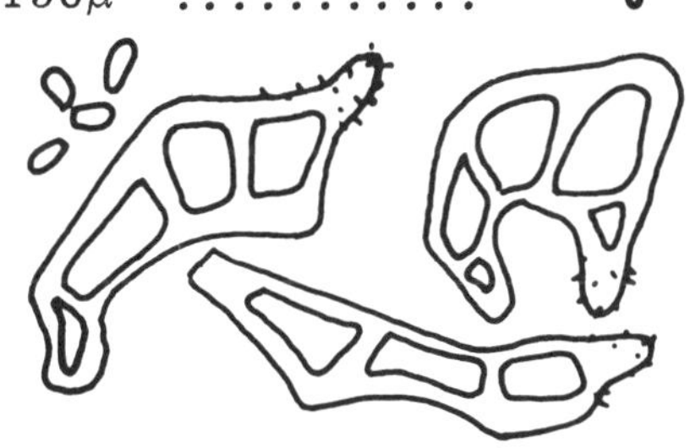

Macroaleuriospores frequently constricted in midlength (hour-glass or tadpole shape) and smooth to densely echinulate, or in excess of 150μ long, fusiform, but with less than 8 cells. Undersurface of thallus colorless or with salmon or peach-tan tints. . . 16 M. audouinii (CHP), rare in animals.

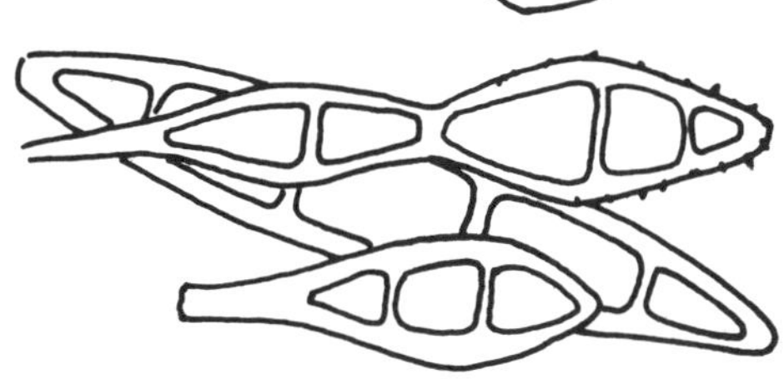

7 Surface of macroaleuriospores more or less echinulate or roughened. Microaleuriospores numerous.................................... 8

Surface of macroaleuriospores entirely smooth. Microaleuriospores usually rare (see photomicrograph 6).................................... 9

8 Macroaleuriospores more or less plump, spindle-shaped, or club-shaped (width usually more than 1/5 the length) echinulate, most containing 7 or less cells. Thallus more or less powdery buff, usually with deep red, non-diffusing pigment beneath the thallus. . . 29 M. cookei (RHP), soil (also check 65 M. amazonicum, and 19 M. ferrugineum).

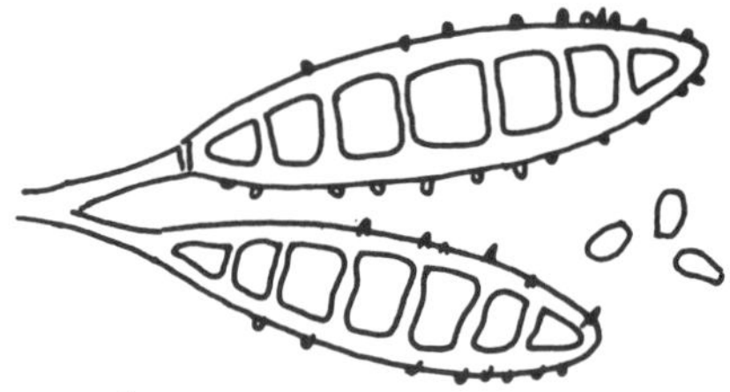

Macroaleuriospores long (width often less than 1/5 the length), cylindrical, or cigar-shaped, frequently containing 8 or more cells and finely echinulate. Microaleuriospores abundant. Surface of thallus powdery cream to pink. . . 30
9 M. vanbreuseghemii (RHP), soil.

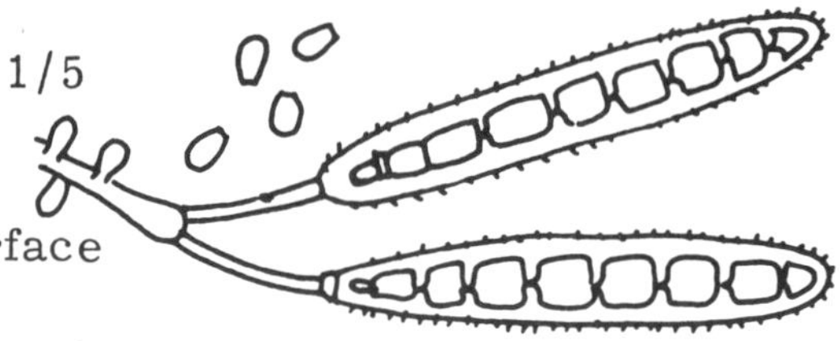

Macroaleuriospores short spindle-shaped, most with 2 - 5 cells. Thallus more or less powdery orange buff. . . 31 T. ajelloi var nana (NHP), soil.

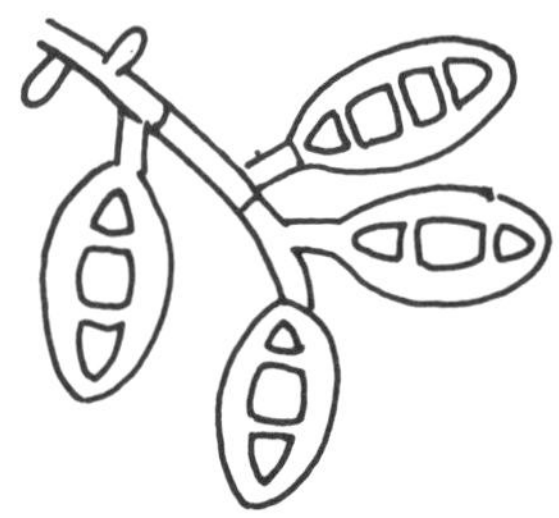

Macroaleuriospores long cylindrical, club-shaped to spindle-shaped, most with 6 or more cells. Microaleuriospores usually rare. Thallus with a more or less rich orange-buff powdery surface, frequently producing purple-black pigment beneath. . . 31 T. ajelloi (NHP), common in soil (also check 30 M. vanbreuseghemii).

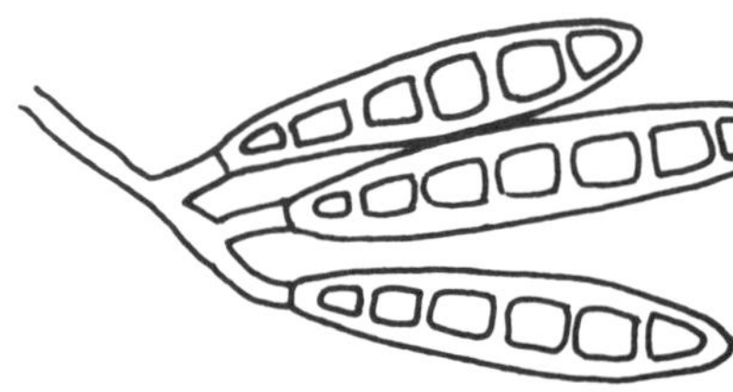

10 Macroaleuriospores spindle-shaped, egg-shaped, club-shaped, or cylindrical, with surface more or less roughened or echinulate, generally more than 7μ in diameter (photomicrographs 7-15) 11

Macroaleuriospores principally club-shaped or cylindrical. Surface not roughened or echinulate, in most cases less than 7μ in diameter if microaleuriospores also present (photomicrographs 16 - 21, 23, 27, 29, 32, 34, 35).. 19

11 Macroaleuriospores egg-shaped or short ellipsoidal most containing 2 cells. Microaleuriospores present (if microaleuriospores are not present, check 71 Chrysosporium). . . 26 M. nanum (RHP), usual in pigs and soil in pigyards.

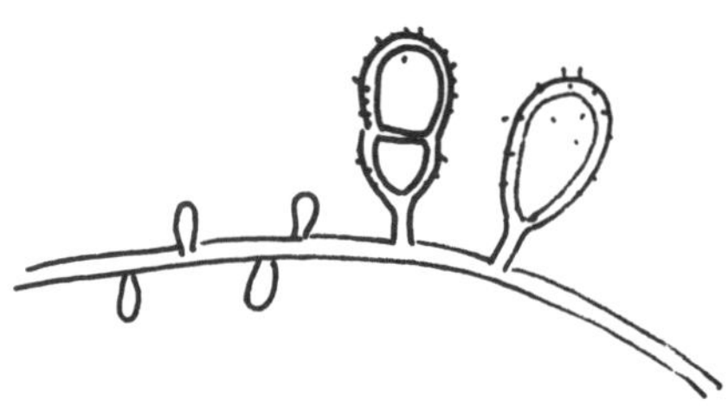

Macroaleuriospores spindle-shaped or elongate, most with more than 3 cells.. 12

12 Macroaleuriospores predominantly spindle-shaped, clavate, club-shaped, bullet-shaped, or cigar-shaped, symmetrical and uncurved, most with 5 or more cells. Attachment scar frequently more than 1/3 the diameter of the macroaleuriospore at its greatest width (photomicrographs 8 - 12) 13

Macroaleuriospores with attachment scar less than 1/3 the diameter of the spore at its greatest width. Macroaleuriospores either (a) spindle-shaped and most containing 4 cells, or (b) fusiform, club-shaped, and tadpole-shaped (frequently curved), with rounded tips, and containing up to 10 cells (photomicrographs 13 and 14)........................... 18

13 Macroaleuriospores spindle-shaped, club-shaped, clavate, bullet-shaped, or cigar-shaped, less than 60μ long, most with 5 to 8 cells or less. Surface of thallus powdery buff to ochre-pink......................... 14

Macroaleuriospores spindle-shaped (not bullet-shaped), frequently more than 60μ long and with more than 6 cells. Surface of thallus buff or powdery cream to grape red...................................... 17

14 Macroaleuriospores mostly spindle-shaped or ellipsoidal with diameter often 1/3 to 1/4 the length, most containing 6 or less cells, sometimes with a slight terminal beak and produced usually in large numbers in clusters along the hyphae and terminally. Entire surface of thallus usually powdery, olive-buff to cinnamon-tan. A nearly glabrous (silky) isolate with few macroaleuriospores has been reported. Also isolates with smooth macroaleuriospores. . . 23 M. gypseum (CHP), common in soil (also check 25 M. fulvum).

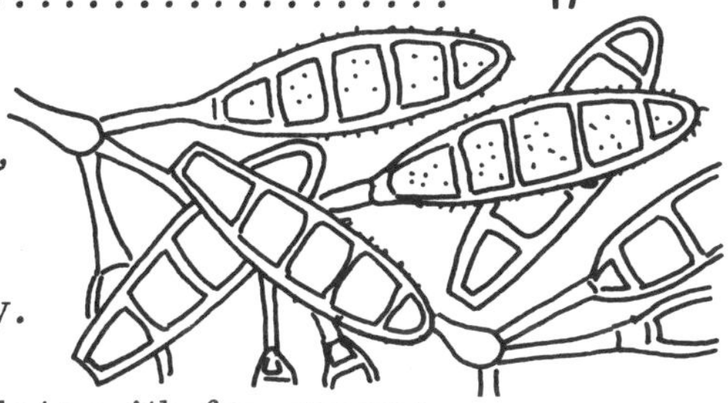

Macroaleuriospores club-shaped, bullet-shaped, cigar-shaped, or spindle-shaped with diameter less than 1/4 the length, most with 6 or more cells, abundant or few, and scattered rather than clustered................ 15

15 Thallus powdery or fluffy, cream color to buff, at times with violet or pink tinted margin. Macroaleuriospores few. Microaleuriospores spherical or club-shaped, in large clusters. Coils frequent. Macroaleuriospores club-shaped and tapered, nearly smooth or else echinulate near the tip. . 26 M. persicolor (RHP), geographically limited to Europe and carried by the Bank Vole (also check 25 M. fulvum, 40 T. mentagrophytes, and 64 M. racemosum).

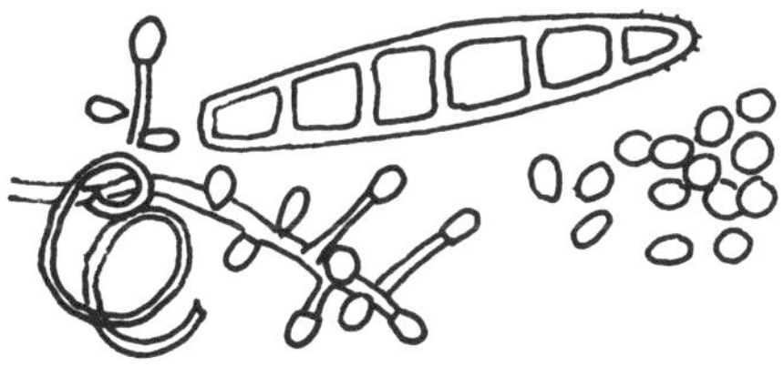

Thallus usually heavily powdery, buff to reddish buff, frequently with a white fluffy border. Macroaleuriospores conspicuously echinulate, usually abundant. Microaleuriospores not in conspicuous clusters, and not the predominant feature....................................... 16

16 Macroaleuriospores thin-walled (photomicrograph 10), mostly less than 50μ in length, club-shaped, spindle-shaped, cigar-shaped, or bullet-shaped, and with 7 or less cells. Thallus buff to reddish buff. . . 25 M. fulvum (RHP), soil (also check 23 M. gypseum and 63 M. boullardii).

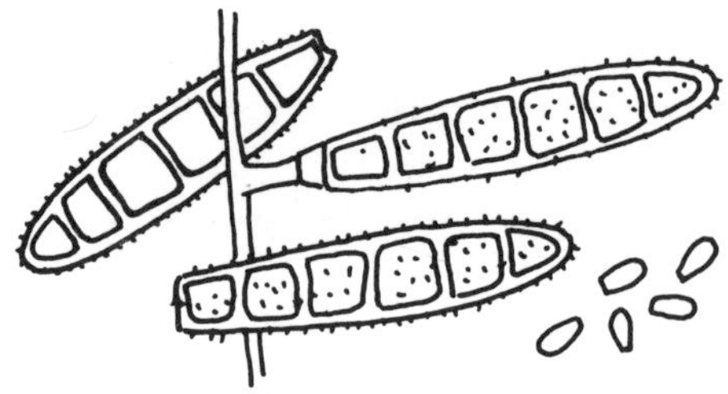

Macroaleuriospores somewhat thick-walled (photomicrograph 11), spindle-shaped, cigar-shaped, or bullet-shaped, frequently with 7 or more cells and frequently achieving length of 50μ or more. Thallus reddish buff. . . 63 M. boullardii (NHP), soil, Africa (also check 25 M. fulvum, 64 M. racemosum, and 64 M. praecox).

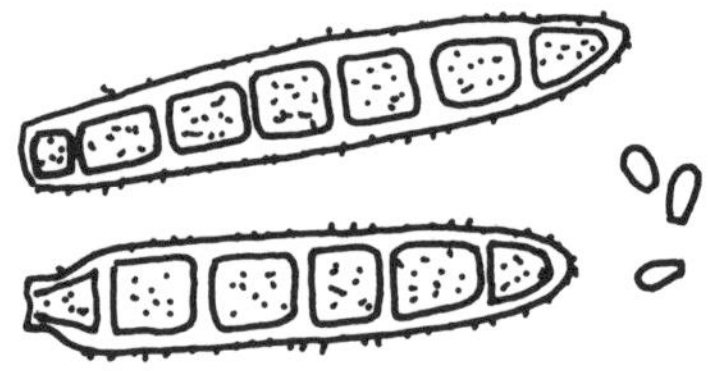

17 Thallus flat, powdery white to cream or stained with grape-red and with dark grape-red undercolor (see Plate IV). Club-shaped microaleuriospores in conspicuous wand-like open terminal clusters (which may be the predominant feature). Macroaleuriospores few to numerous, spindle-shaped, varying in length to over 60μ, and with 5 to 10 cells. . . 64 M. racemosum (NHP), soil.

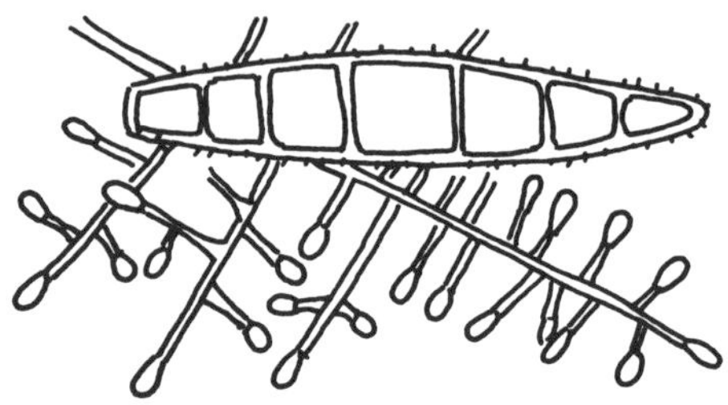

Surface of thallus powdery buff. Undersurface yellow-orange. Microaleuriospores not in conspicuous clusters. Macroaleuriospores slender spindle-shaped, many over 60μ long, and with up to 9 cells. . . 64 M. praecox (RHP) (also check 23 M. gypseum, 25 M. fulvum, and 62 M. boullardii).

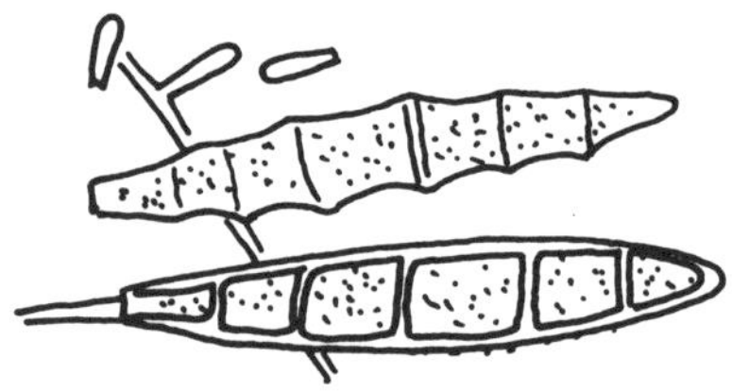

18 Thallus olive-buff to olive-grey, fluffy to heavily powdery. Macroaleuriospores containing up to 7 or more cells, but most with only 4 cells and short, symmetrical, spindle-shaped, with both cell walls and septa frequently thickened, and frequently containing oil drop-like inclusion in each cell (photomicrograph 13). Attachment scar small, usually less than 1/5 diameter of the aleuriospore at its greatest width. . . 65 M. amazonicum (NHP), soil, Brazil (also check 23 M. gypseum).

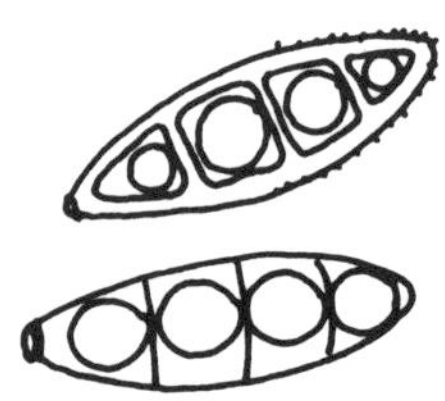

Thallus usually white to pink white or brown, satiny to fluffy, rarely powdery buff. Macroaleuriospores slightly echinulate or smooth, blunt-tipped, frequently tadpole shaped and curved, containing up to 10 cells, and frequently on comb-like hyphal branches (photomicrograph 14). Attachment scar usually less than 1/3 diameter of the spore at its greatest width. A diffusing yellow to strawberry red pigment usually produced beneath the thallus. . . 21 *T. (M?) gallinae* (RHP), chicken (also check *29 M. cookei*).

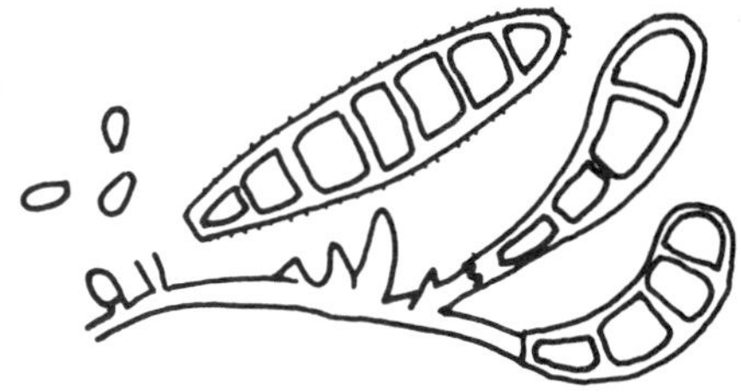

19 Macroaleuriospores and attachment scar usually less than 1/3 the diameter of the spore at its greatest width. Macroaleuriospores blunt-tipped, spindle-shaped, club-shaped, or tadpole-shaped, frequently curved (photomicrograph 14). Microaleuriospores usually present. Mature thallus usually developing a yellow to strawberry red diffusing pigment. . . 21 *T. (M?) gallinae* (RHP), chicken.

Macroaleuriospores with attachment scar in most cases more than 1/3 the diameter of the spore at its greatest width, if not then microaleuriospores absent. Macroaleuriospores generally thin-walled, club-shaped, or cylindrical. Strawberry red diffusing pigment rarely produced..... 20

20 Microaleuriospores present and predominantly cashew nut-shaped (photomicrograph 24), and produced laterally or abundantly in ascocarp-like structures composed of thickened hyphae (pycnidia) . . . 66 *T. phaseoliforme* (NHP), soil (also check 27 *M. persicolor*).

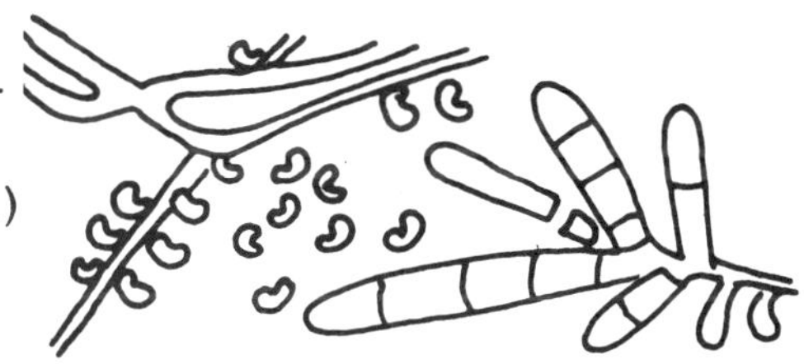

Microaleuriospores absent, or if present not predominantly cashew nut-shaped or curved, and rarely in ascocarp-like structures........... 21

21 Microaleuriospores (small, one-celled aleuriospores) absent; or macroaleuriospores usually large, frequently more than 9μ in diameter or more than 100μ long. 22

Microaleuriospores (small, one-celled aleuriospores) present. Macroaleuriospores usually less than 9μ in diameter and less than 100μ long. 23

22 Macroaleuriospores large, cylindrical (usually more than 9μ in diameter) and produced on slender stalks. Attachment scar may be less than 1/3 the diameter of the spore at its greatest width. Thallus flat, white to buff, frequently with concentric rings of growth, and yellow underneath. . . 70 *A. flavescens* (NHP), from feathers of Australian birds.

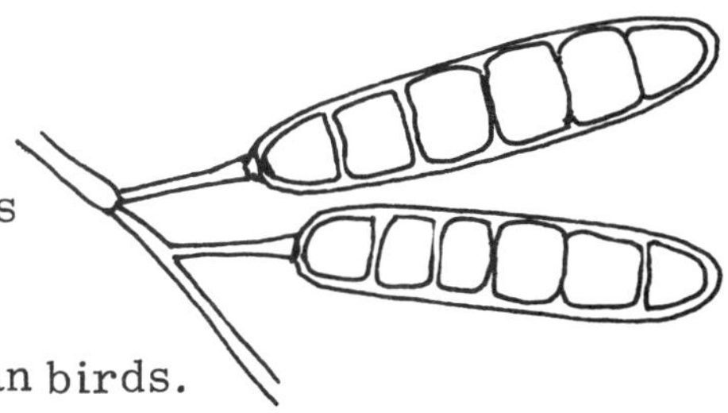

Macroaleuriospores club-shaped or cylindrical and attached together and joined in groups (photomicrographs 16 and 21)................... 23

23 Macroaleuriospores blunt, club-shaped, frequently more than 7μ in diameter, and attached together in groups. Thallus usually mustard or khaki color, with rough or folded surface. . . .62 E. floccosum (CHP), principally tinea cruris and pedis (also check 33 T. terrestre, 31 T. ajelloi, and 50 T. rubrum).

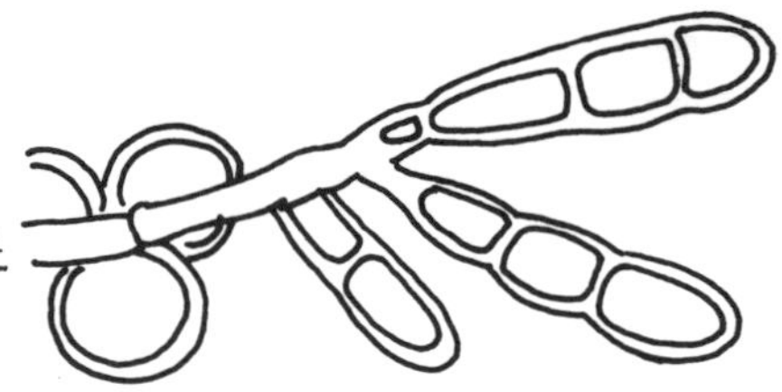

Macroaleuriospores elongate, cylindrical, and frequently attached together. Thallus flat and powdery, yellowish or cream-white to tan. . 67 T. longifusus (NHP), soil.

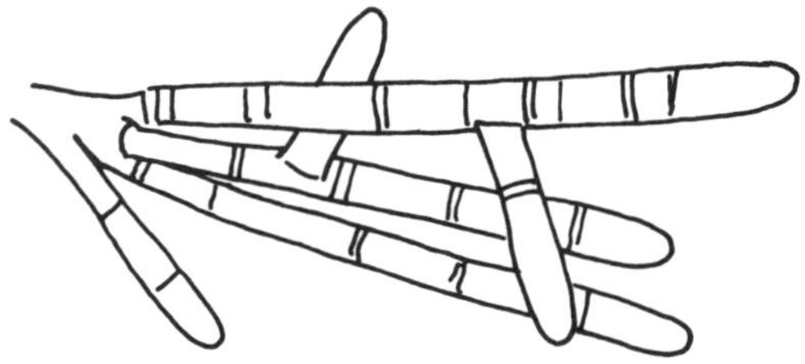

24 Macroaleuriospores narrow (usually less than 7μ in diameter) principally born laterally or terminally, not markedly differentiated from lateral clavate, one-celled microaleuriospores (photomicrographs 23, 29, 32). 25

Macroaleuriospores narrow as above, or thick (more than 7μ in diameter) and born singly or in groups, sometimes with "microaleuriospore-like" one-celled elements, but clearly differentiated from the small, more or less spherical, club-shaped, or teardrop-shaped microaleuriospores... 29

25 Macroaleuriospores principally terminal or lateral on slender stalks, and when attached tapering toward the base; pencil-shaped, spindle-shaped, or club-shaped when detached, and sometimes appearing slightly roughened (photomicrograph 24). "Propagules" present in the depths of the thallus . . .67 T. proliferans (RHP), ecology unknown (also check 44 T. erinacei, 27 M. persicolor, and 50 T. rubrum).

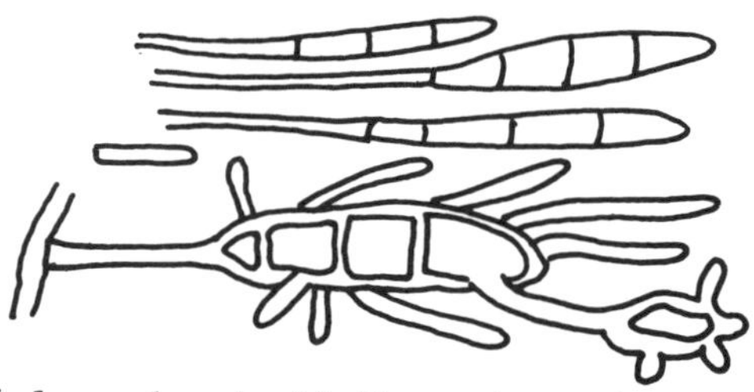

Macroaleuriospores predominantly lateral, club-shaped, or cylindrical, scattered or in terminal clusters, and not tapering toward the base when attached (photomicrographs 23 and 29)............................ 26

26 Thallus reddish or reddish-brown.................................... 27

Thallus white, yellowish, greenish, or cinnamon buff................ 28

27 Macroaleuriospores frequently long cylindrical or tapered (exceeding 40μ) and frequently forming terminal filaments while still attached to the hyphae. Mature thallus frequently developing a cracked surface. . . . 27 T. fluviomuniense (RHP), ecology unknown (also check 33 T. terrestre, 52 T. tonsurans, 49 T. megninii, 50 T. rubrum, and 40 T. mentagrophytes).

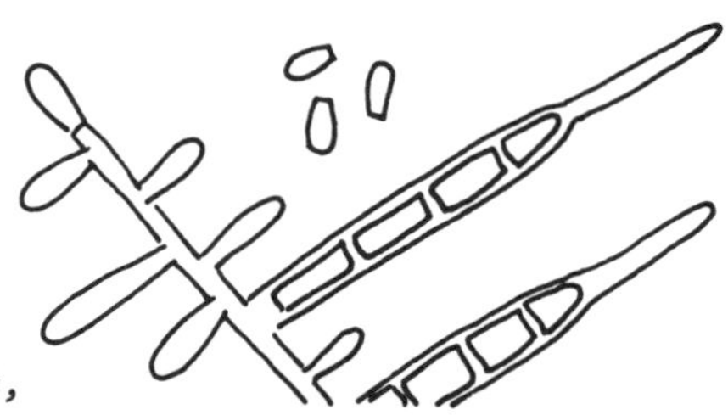

Macroaleuriospores predominantly small and cylindrical, usually less than 6 X 40μ, and not forming terminal germ tubes before detachment . . . 33 T. terrestre, 68 T. thuringiense, etc. (NHP), soil. Separations largely depend on demonstrating the perfect states. T. terrestre may produce diffusing red pigment (also check 69 T. fluviomuniense, 35 T. georgiae, and 44 T. erinacei).

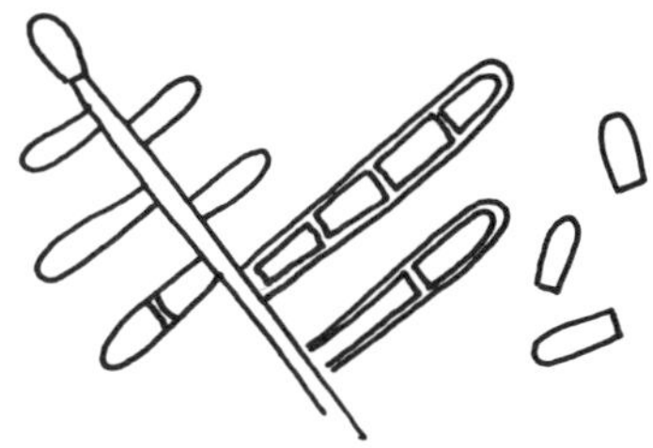

28 Thallus white, yellowish, or greenish. Smallest mature, detached, one-celled elements (microaleuriospores) predominantly large and clavate (most more than 1.5 X 3μ) (photomicrographs 29). Lateral macroaleuriospores not conspicuously clustered terminally, but scattered more or less evenly throughout the aerial hyphae. . . 33 T. terrestre, 70 A. cuniculi, etc. (NHP), soil. Separations largely depend on demonstrating the perfect states.

Thallus white, yellowish, or cinnamon buff. Smallest mature, detached microaleuriospores usually small and tear-drop shaped or elongate (less than 1.5 X 3μ). Lateral macroaleuriospores usually conspicuously clustered terminally in groups of up to 50 macroaleuriospores (photomicrographs 23 and 34). . . 36 T. gloriae (NHP), soil (also check 49 T. rubrum and 38 T. simii).

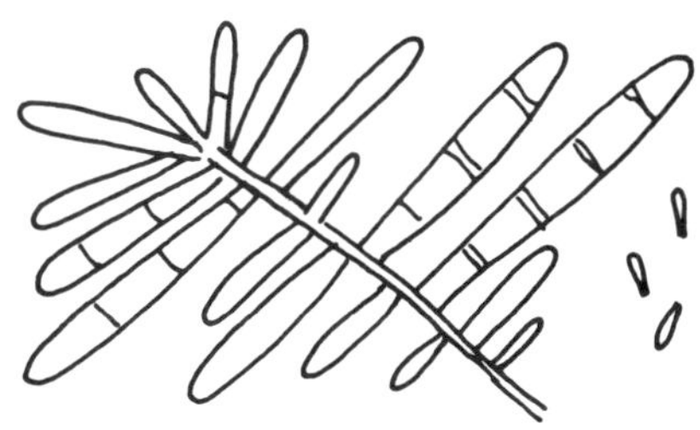

29 Macroaleuriospores remaining a conspicuous and abundant feature in maturing thallus. Microaleuriospores predominantly or exclusively lateral on non-terminal hyphae or on terminal hyphal branches. **30**

Microaleuriospores a more conspicuous feature in maturing thallus than macroaleuriospores and either lateral on non-terminal hyphae or terminal hyphal branches; or in conspicuous branched and unbranched terminal clusters; or on thickened terminal or subterminal hyphae (photomicrographs 25, 26, 27, 33, 36); or both macroaleuriospores and microaleuriospores rare. . . **41**

30 Macroaleuriospores narrow (most less than 7μ in diameter), the largest usually appearing long, cylindrical, or fragmented, length frequently more than 7 times diameter (photomicrographs 23, 34, 35). **31**

Macroaleuriospores frequently 7μ in diameter or larger, the largest usually appearing well-formed, and club-shaped, narrow fusiform or short, cylindrical, length usually less than 7 times the diameter (photomicrographs 17, 18, 19). **33**

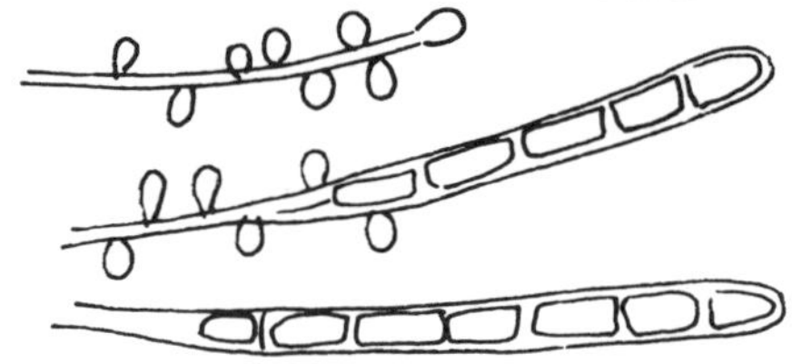

31 Macroaleuriospores narrow, long, cylindrical, mainly terminal, sometimes poorly differentiated from thickened hyphae tips or arthrospores, but well differentiated from egg-shaped to peg-shaped or short club-shaped lateral microaleuriospores. Microaleuriospores sometimes produced laterally on the macroaleuriospores. Thallus usually purplish red beneath and with a fluffy or more or less heaped and glabrous surface. . . 50 T. rubrum (CHP), principally tinea corporis, tinea pedis and tinea manus (also check 38 T. simii and 23 M. gypseum).

Macroaleuriospores narrow, varying in length from short one-celled and microaleuriospore-like to long cylindrical, with up to 10 cells, and produced mostly laterally along the hyphae or in terminal clusters............ 32

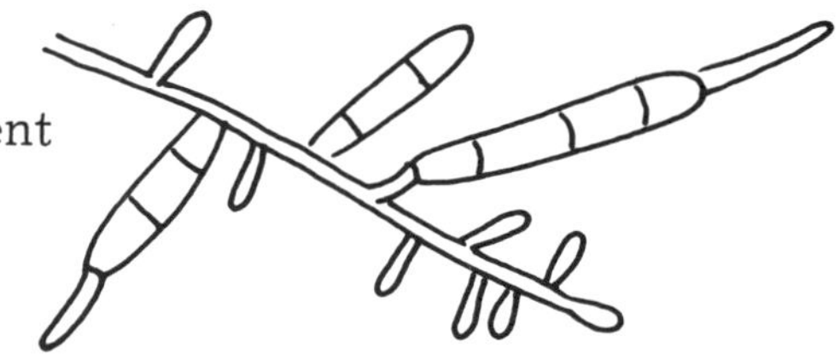

32 Macroaleuriospores, frequently with terminal filaments produced laterally, but not in conspicuous clusters. Smallest microaleuriospore elements short clavate (about 3 X 5.5) with broad attachment scars. Surface of thallus granular, folded, and cracked, and red-brown in color. . .69 T. fluviomuniense (RHP), ecology unknown (also check 33 T. terrestre, 52 T. tonsurans, 49 T. megninii, 50 T. rubrum, 40 T. mentagrophytes, and 23 M. gypseum).

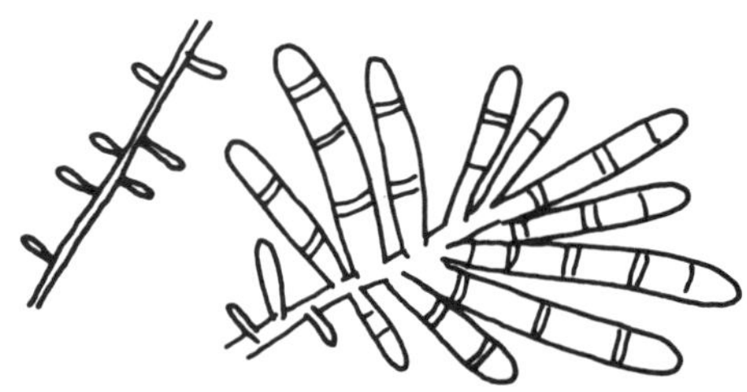

Macroaleuriospores without frequent terminal germ tubes and produced laterally in terminal clusters of up to 50 (photomicrograph 23). Small tear-drop shaped microaleuriospores (about 1.5 X 3μ) also present (photomicrograph 34). Surface of thallus more or less powdery, flat, and yellowish to cinnamon; yellow beneath. Arthroaleuriospores may be frequent. . .36 T. gloriae (NHP), soil (also check 27 M. persicolor, 33 T. terrestre, and 50 T. rubrum).

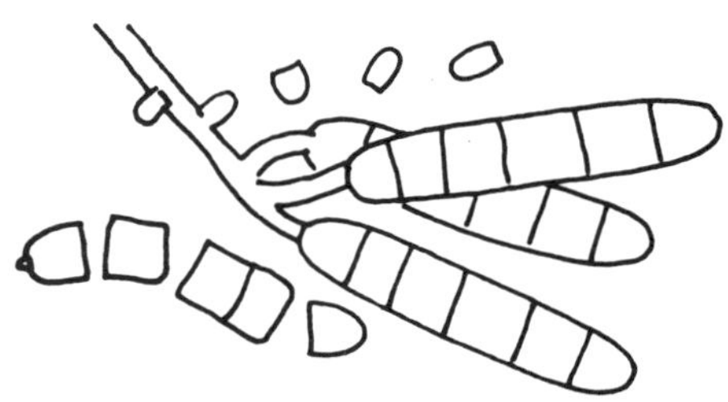

33 Macroaleuriospores blunt, cylindrical, and thick (7 to 10μ in diameter), most of relatively uniform length or varying in length from one-celled to larger elements, and produced terminally and laterally in small clusters or in masses. Cells of macroaleuriospores frequently disarticulating when mature (photomicrograph 17). Surface of thallus cream to cream buff . . .37 T. vanbreuseghemii (RHP), soil (also check 38 T. simii, 36 T. gloriae, 40 T. mentagrophytes, and 23 M. gypseum).

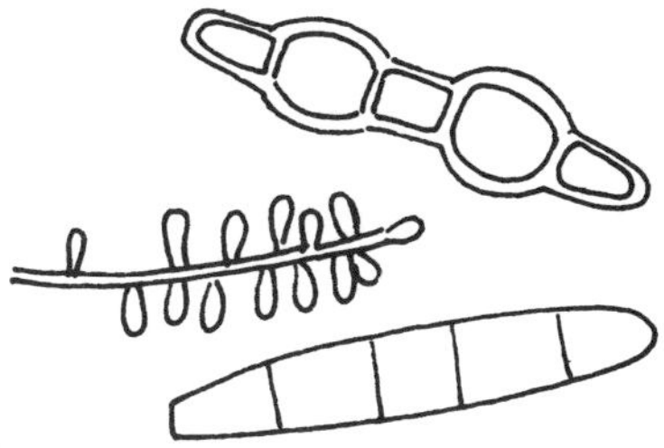

Macroaleuriospores tapered and club-shaped to long cylindrical, frequently developing distinctive swollen cells when mature (photomicrograph 18). Macroaleuriospores frequently clustered or massed in large numbers. Microaleuriospores clavate to teardrop-shaped, sometimes with slender bases or stalks, and produced laterally on non-terminal hyphal branches. Surface of thallus powdery white to cream or reddish. Undersurface usually yellow to reddish. . . 38 T. simii (RHP), monkey, chicken, and soil, restricted to penisular India (also check 40 T. mentagrophytes, 36 T. vanbreuseghemii, 44 T. erinacei, and 50 T. rubrum).

34 Microaleuriospores (predominantly one celled) present............... 35

Neither macroaleuriospores nor microaleuriospores present......... 48

35 Microaleuriospores frequently or predominantly cashew nut-shaped (photomicrograph 24) and frequently produced in ascocarp-like structures (pycnidia). . . 66 T. phaseoliforme (NHP), soil (also check 27 M. persicolor).

Microaleuriospores not predominantly cashew nut-shaped and rarely produced in ascocarp-like structures................................. 36

36 Microaleuriospores mostly large (more than 7μ long) egg-shaped, spherical, or ellipsoidal, predominantly with one cell, but approaching in size and shape the macroaleuriospores of M. nanum (photomicrograph 30)...... 37

Microaleuriospores mostly small (less than 7μ long) spherical, pear-shaped, egg-shaped, club-shaped, or oat-shaped............................ 38

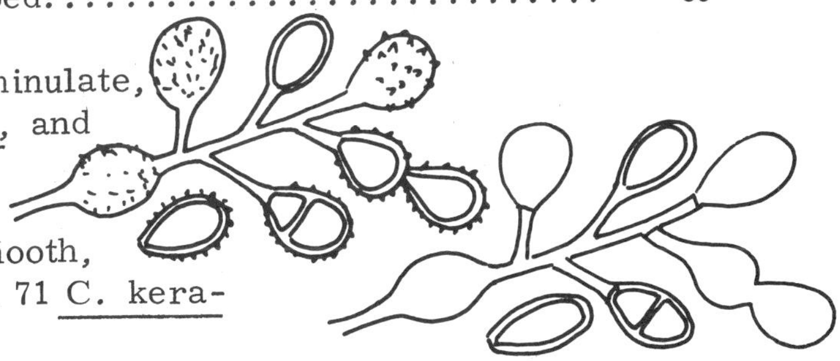

37 Microaleuriospores predominantly echinulate, 70 A. tuberculatum, 71 C. asperatum, and 71 C. serratus (NHP), soil.

Microaleuriospores predominantly smooth, 70 A. multifidum, 70 A. curreyi, and 71 C. keratinophilum (NHP), soil.

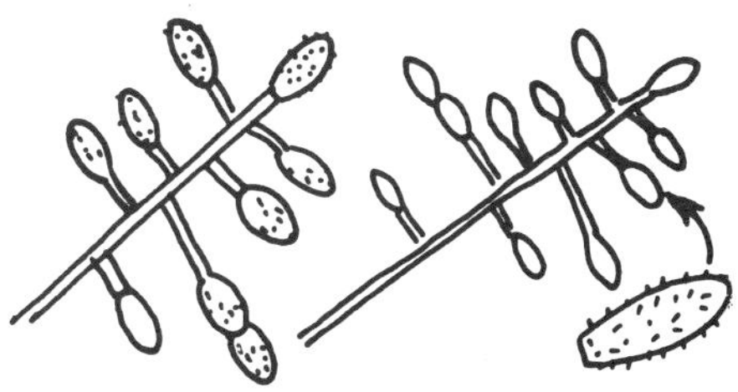

38 Microaleuriospores more or less oat-shaped, surface finely echinulate. No macroaleuriospores produced (photomicrograph 22). Surface of thallus powdery white to cream. . . 71 C. indicum and 71 C. evolceanui (NHP), soil (differentiate by size and perfect state).

Microaleuriospores with smooth surface and generally spherical, club-shaped, egg-shaped, teardrop-shaped, etc......................... 39

39 Microaleuriospores frequently on long lateral stalks (more than 2X the length of microaleuriospores) or frequently in chains of two or more (photomicrographs 28 and 31), and scattered more or less abundantly throughout the surface branches in the thallus, but not conspicuously or predominantly in branched terminal clusters or on thickened terminal or subterminal hyphae (photomicrographs 28 and 31). No macroaleuriospores produced... .... **40**

Microaleuriospores not conspicuously on long stalks or in chains; or if on stalks, stalks less than 2X the length of the microaleuriospores; or microaleuriospores conspicuously in more or less branched terminal clusters or cluster-like masses, or on thickened terminal or subterminal hyphae (photomicrographs 25, 26, 27, 33, 36)...................... **41**

40 Microaleuriospores rarely in chains of two or more (catenulate). Microaleuriospores club-shaped, small, less than 2.5 X 4.5μ. Thallus rosy buff, loosely powdery, and slightly domed (see Plate IV). . . .35 T. georgiae (NHP), soil (also check 71 C. pannorum).

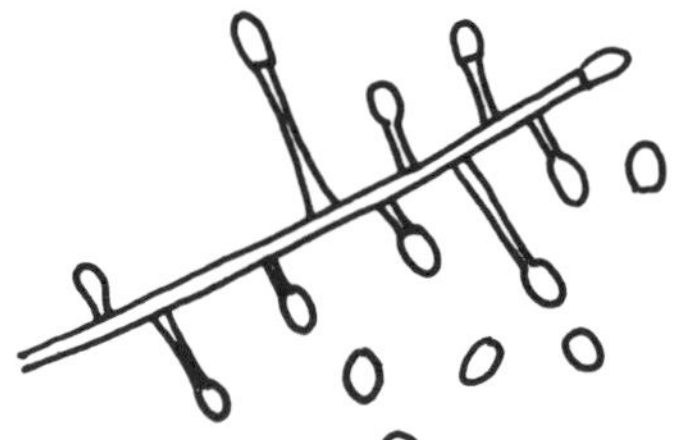

Microaleuriospores club-shaped, oat-shaped, and egg-shaped, sometimes in chains of 2 or more (catenulate) and large (3.5 X 8μ or more). Thallus white to cream-color usually flat and powdery . . . .71 C. tropicum (NHP), soil (also check 71 C. evolceanui, 71 C. indicum, 71 C. pannorum, 72 C. pruinosum, and 33 T. terrestre).

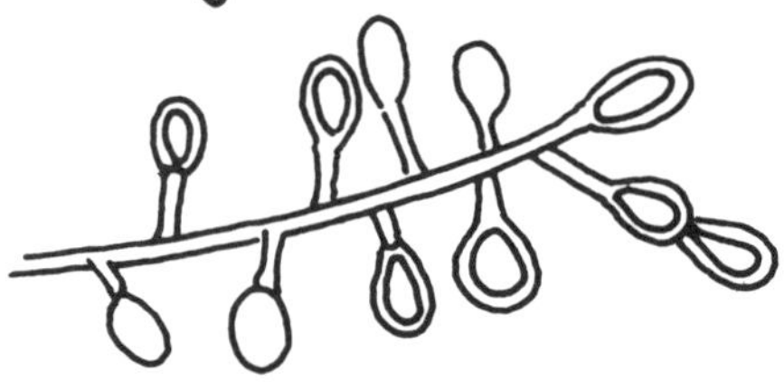

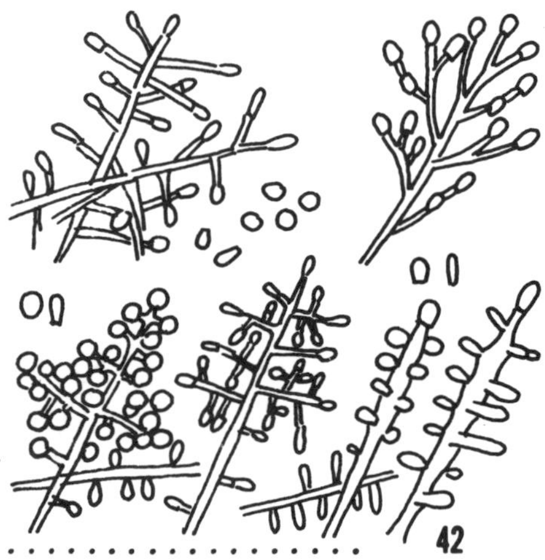

41 Microaleuriospores usually numerous in more or less conspicuous, variously branched, terminal clusters, or on thickened terminal hyphae, and in some cases differing in size and shape from those produced laterally on non-terminal hyphae. Microaleuriospores in some cases predominantly spherical (photomicrographs 25, 26, 27, 33). **42**

Microaleuriospores few to numerous, mainly lateral on non-terminal hyphae, or clustered on undifferentiated terminal hyphal branches. Microaleuriospores clustered terminally not differing conspicuously in size and shape from those produced laterally on non-terminal hyphae, and not predominantly spherical.. **48**

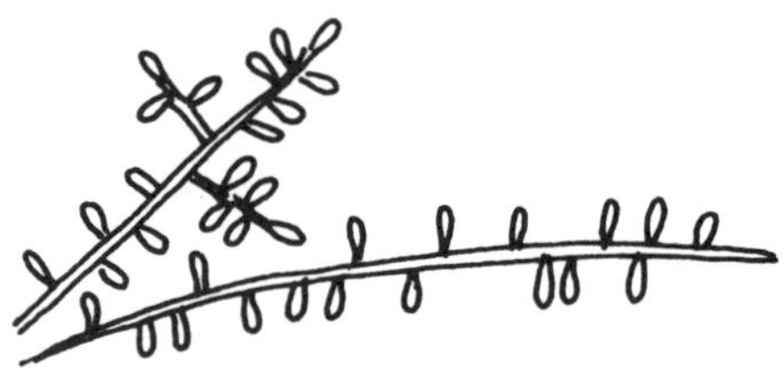

42 Microaleuriospores in conspicuous branched clusters in the mature thallus and predominantly spherical when mature and detached. Macroaleuriospores and spiral hyphae often present.. **43**

Microaleuriospores in branched clusters or not, but predominantly club-shaped, teardrop-shaped, or peg-shaped when mature and detached... **44**

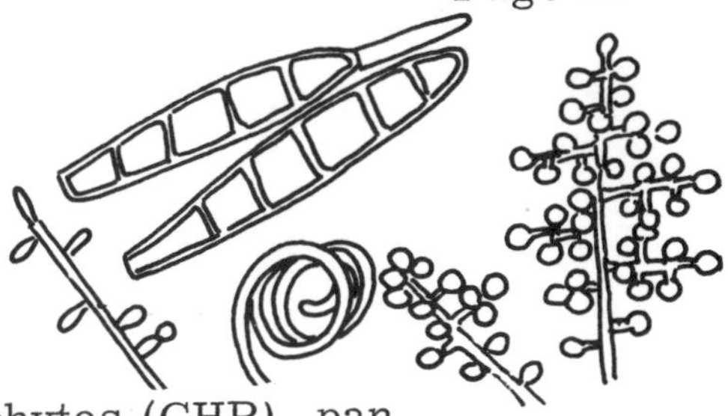

43 Immature microaleuriospores in clusters in primary culture or subculture mostly not stalked and frequently spherical (photomicrograph 25). Macroaleuriospores few to numerous, club-shaped usually with 4 or more cells. Lateral microaleuriospores usually more teardrop-shaped. Spiral hyphae often present. . . 40 T. mentagrophytes (CHP), pan zoophilic, principally tinea pedis, and tinea corporis (photomicrograph 19) (also check 52 T. tonsurans and 27 M. persicolor).

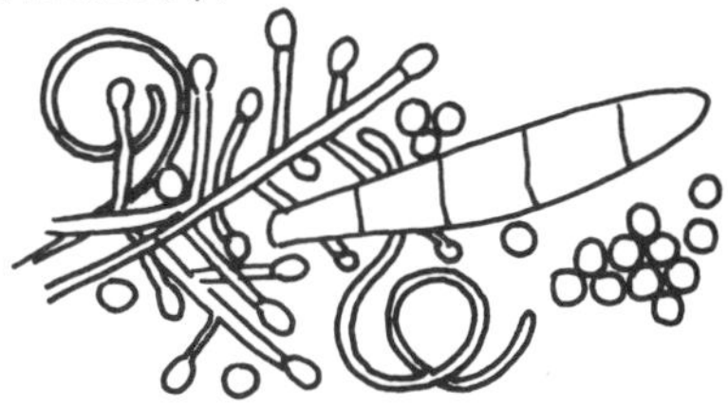

Immature microaleuriospores in clusters frequently on long stalks (stalks more than 3X of the length of microaleuriospores) and club-shaped (photomicrograph 33). Macroaleuriospores usually scattered and club-shaped or somewhat spindle shaped (photomicrograph 9). Spiral hyphae often present. . . 27 M. persicolor (RHP), geographically limited to Europe and carried by the Bank Vole (also check 40 T. mentagrophytes, 25 M. fulvum, and 52 T. tonsurans).

44 Microaleuriospores in clusters, or on thickened hyphae, frequently on long stalks (stalks more than 3X length of microaleuriospores)....... **45**

Microaleuriospores in clusters, or on thickened hyphae, mostly not on long stalks (stalks, if present less than 3X length of microaleuriospores). **47**

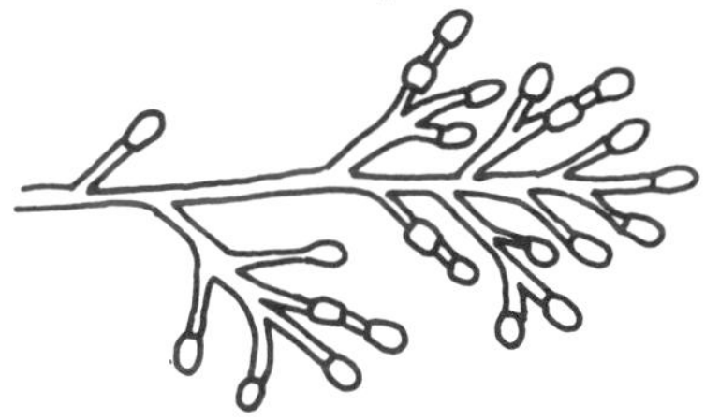

45 Microaleuriospores in clusters conspicuously on forward-directed branches and stalks and produced singly or in chains of two or more. No macroaleuriospores produced. . . 71 C. pannorum (NHP), soil (also check 71 C. tropicum).

Microaleuriospores in clusters not conspicuously on forward directed branches and stalks. Chains of aleuriospores rare or absent......... **46**

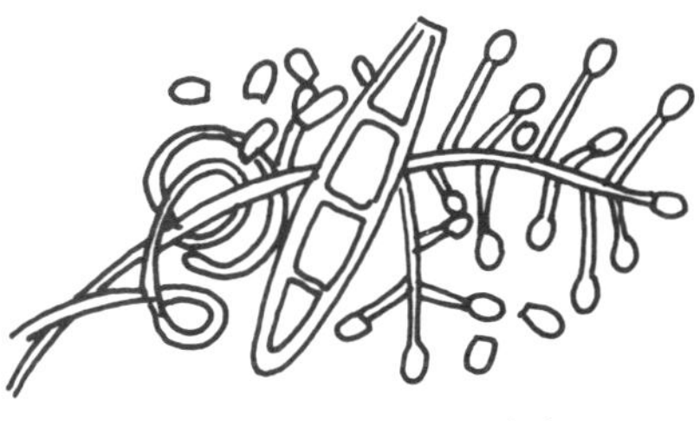

46 Microaleuriospores usually in large twiggy clusters or masses and usually or relatively uniform size and shape (photomicrograph 33). Macroaleuriospores usually present and well formed and tapered or club-shaped (photomicrograph 9). Thallus fluffy to densely powdery, cream-buff, frequently developing pink tints. . . 27 M. persicolor (RHP), geographically limited to Europe and carried by the Bank Vole (also check 40 T. mentagrophytes).

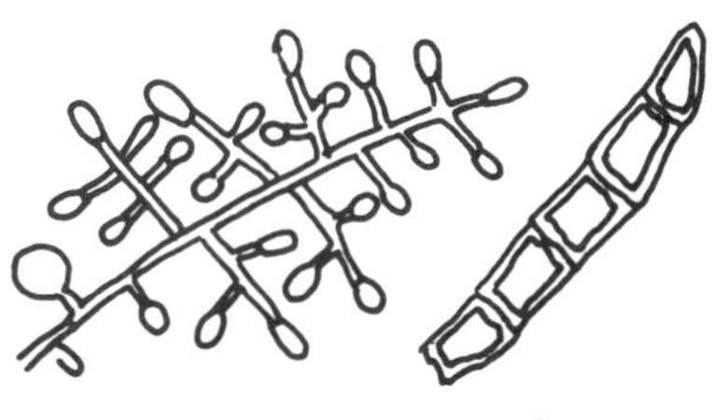

Microaleuriospores of variable size and shape, predominantly club-shaped, long club-shaped, or filiform, frequently lateral on thickened terminal hyphae (photomicrograph 26), and in clusters usually of twiggy aspect, and frequently with spherical balloon forms. Macroaleuriospores usually rare and short cylindrical or poorly formed. Young thallus slightly powdery, mature thallus suede-like and flat or folded. Undersurface of thallus mahogany brown, yellow, or colorless. . . 52 T. tonsurans (CHP) primarily endothrix scalp ringworm (also check 40 T. mentagrophytes).

47 Microaleuriospores of variable size and shape, frequently stalked, predominantly long, club-shaped, or filiform, and frequently lateral on thickened terminal hyphae (photomicrograph 26) and in clusters usually of twiggy aspect, and frequently developing into spherical balloon forms. Macroaleuriospores usually rare and short cylindrical or poorly formed (length less than 6 times diameter). Undersurface of thallus mahogany brown, yellow, or colorless. . . 52 T. tonsurans (CHP), primarily endothrix scalp ringworm (also check 50 T. rubrum).

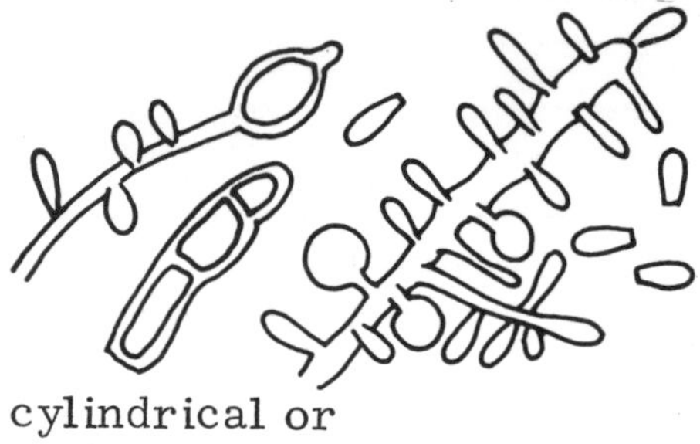

Microaleuriospores in clusters or on thickened terminal hyphae, and often short club-shaped, or plump, frequently with attachment scars more than 1/2 the length of the spore. Lateral microaleuriospores on non-terminal hyphae frequently small and peg-shaped with attachment scar less than 1/3 the length of the spore. Filiform microaleuriospores not a predominant feature. Spherical balloon forms sometimes present. Thickened terminal hyphae bearing lateral microaleuriospores may be present, or microaleuriospores may be born directly on the basal portion of macroaleuriospores. Macroaleuriospores usually present and frequently long, cylindrical, length more than 7 times diameter, or if thicker frequently fragmented into segments. Microaleuriospores on stalks infrequent (photomicrograph 27). Undersurface of thallus frequently becoming venous blood color with maturity, rarely yellow or brown. . . 50 T. rubrum (CHP), mostly tinea corporis and tinea pedis (also check 49 T. megninii and 52 T. tonsurans).

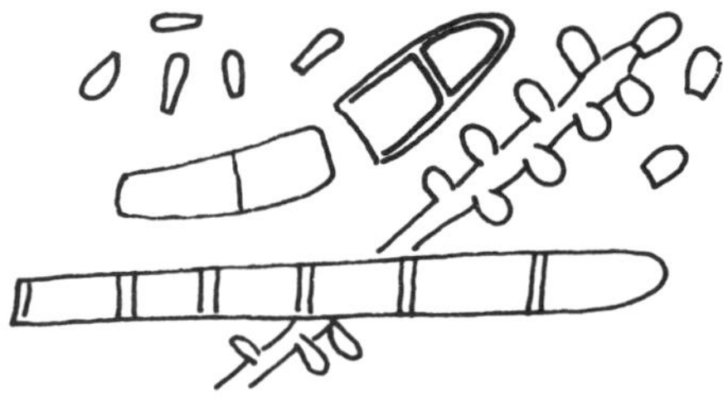

48 Thallus glabrous and heaped up, waxy, verrucose, or convoluted - See Color Plates I(16, 19); II(47); III(50, 54, 56, 58, 59, 61); IV(40). **49**

Thallus downy to fluffy, and flat or folded; or powdery - See Color Plates I(13, 16); II(40, 44, 45, 49); III(50, 52); IV(13, 16, 40, 52). **64**

49 Thallus red, purple, or yellow. **50**

Thallus white or brown. **59**

50 Thallus red or purple. **51**

Thallus yellow to orange. **53**

51 Mycelia usually with abundant disconnected hyphal segments and elongate macroaleuriospores or fragments of macroaleuriospores. More or less fluffy mutants with abundant microaleuriospores commonly appear. Only slight enhancement of growth with the thiamine. . . 50 T. rubrum (CHP), usually from tinea corporis, tinea pedis, and tinea manus (also check 54 T. violaceum, 55 T. gourvilii, and 56 T. soudanense).

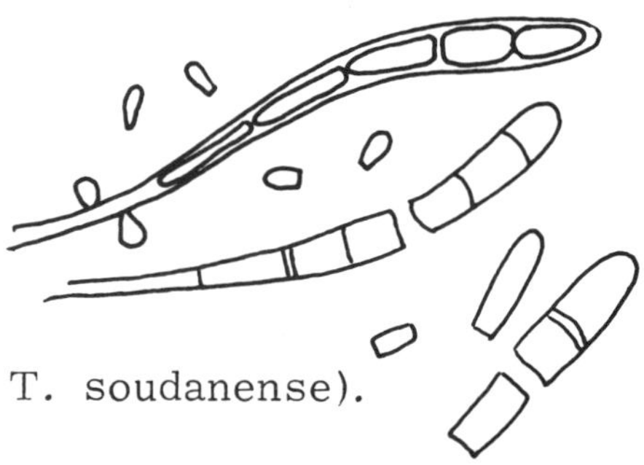

Mycelia without abundant arthrospores. Macroaleuriospores few or absent. Commonly from endothrix tinea capitis.................... 52

52 Thallus waxy or verrucose, and usually dark purplish red. Mycelia much branched and entangled, usually without abundant arthrospores and without aleuriospores. Microaleuriospores rarely or never produced. Not commonly mutating to aleuriospore producing types. Requiring thiamine for growth . . . 54 T. violaceum (CHP), principally endothrix tinea capitis (also check 55 T. gourvilii, 49 T. rubrum, and 56 T. soudanense).

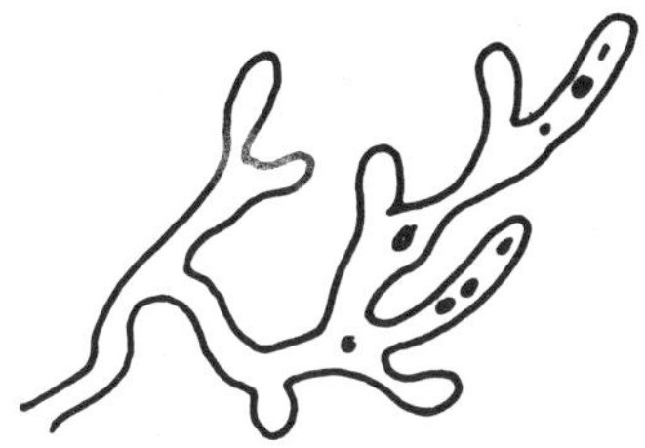

Thallus purplish red or garnet red, glabrous to slightly fluffy, frequently centrally accuminate with a flat radiating border. Microaleuriospores often present. Macroaleuriospores short, club-shaped, and infrequent. Not requiring thiamine . . . 55 T. gourvilii (CHP), principally endothrix tinea capitis. Geographically localized in equatorial and west Africa (also check 56 T. soundanense, 54 T. violaceum, 50 T. rubrum, and 49 T. megninii).

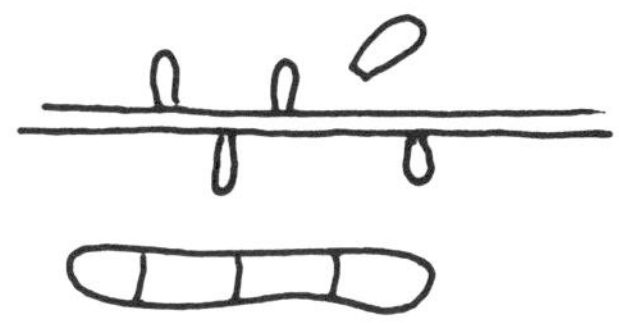

53 Culture producing frequent nodular organs or regularly developing a fluffy perimeter - Plate I(40), with microaleuriospores suggestive of T. mentagrophytes; or mutating to fuzzy violet type - Plate III(50), with macro- and microaleuriospores typical of T. rubrum............... 54

Macro- and microaleuriospores usually rare or absent. Culture not producing frequent nodular organs or regularly developing a fluffy perimeter and microaleuriospores suggestive of T. mentagrophytes; or not mutating to fuzzy violet type of T. rubrum......................... 55

54 Culture usually mutating to fuzzy violet type with microscopic features of T. rubrum (elongate macroaleuriospores and tear-shaped microaleuriospores, see item 50). . . 50 T. rubrum (CHP), principally tinea corporis and tinea pedis (also check 56 T. soudanense and 55 T. gourvilii).

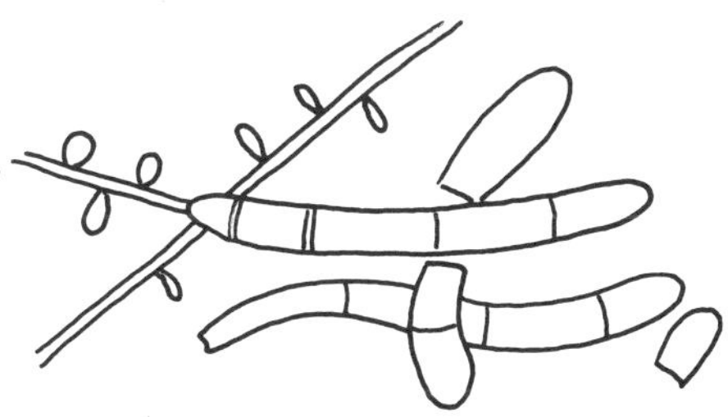

Mycelia with frequent nodular organs. Arthrospores may be present. Thallus usually developing a fluffy pleomorphic perimeter in about one week, and with spherical or tear-shaped microaleuriospores and other structures suggestive of T. mentagrophytes . . . 40 T. mentagrophytes var. nodulare (CHP), principally tinea pedis (also check 62 E. floccosum, 13 M. canis and 52 T. tonsurans).

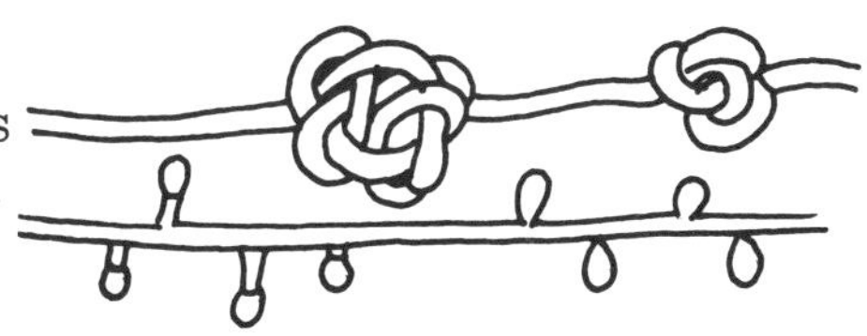

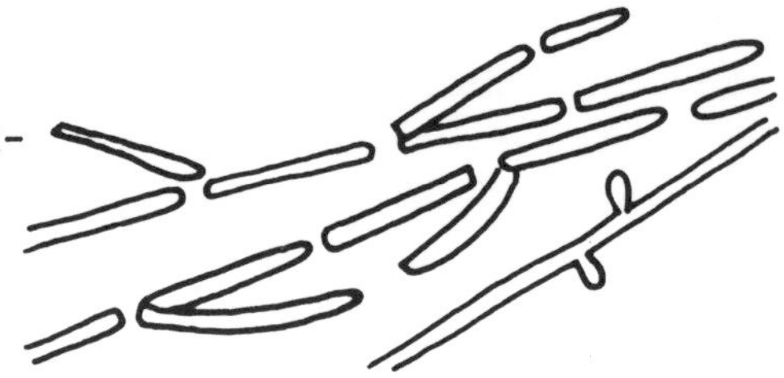

55 Thallus glabrous to slightly fluffy, heaped or centrally accuminate, frequently with a conspicuously fringed perimeter - Plate III(56). Hyphae and abundant arthrospores in brush-like bundles and with frequent reflexive branching. Microaleuriospores sometimes present. . .
56 T. soudanense (CHP), principally tinea capitis, rare outside of equatorial Africa (also check 19 M. ferrugineum, 50 T. rubrum, 13 M. canis, and 46 T. verrucosum).

Reflexive branching not present. Thallus glabrous to slightly fluffy, and heaped, centrally accuminate, cerebriform, submerged, or spreading and with radial grooves. Perimeter of thallus irregular, submerged, sometimes more or less fringed - Plates I(19); II(47); III(61). Arthrospores or disarticulated, clubbed hyphae may be present, but not in brush-like bundles; or hyphae mainly branched and clubbed with frequent chalmydospores. 56

56 Thallus yellow-orange to rust-colored, heaped and slow growing, or spreading. Mycelium irregular, swollen and fragmented, or straight with or without terminal branching, but not highly branched throughout. Subcultured thallus retaining these features, or becoming coarse, fluffy, with hyphae straight and relatively unbranched. Frequently associated with ectothrix, fluorescent tinea capitis.............................. 57

Initial or subcultured thallus yellow or orange, without fragmented hyphae as a predominant feature. Mycelia consisting predominantly of a mass of irregular, antler-like, frequently clubbed branches and chlamydospores. Mainly associated with inflammatory tinea capitis, tinea corporis, tinea barbae, or favus, or tokelau................... 58

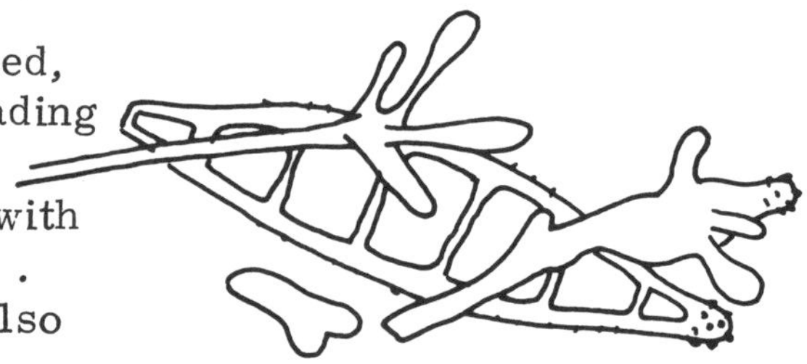

57 Often converting in a week or so from fragmented, swollen mycelia to typical M. canis, with spreading fluffy thallus and fusiform macroaleuriospores (see item 4), or else growth poor and limited, with production of abortive terminal branching. . .
13 M. canis disgonic forms (CHP), zoophilic (also check 19 M. ferrugineum and 52 T. tonsurans).

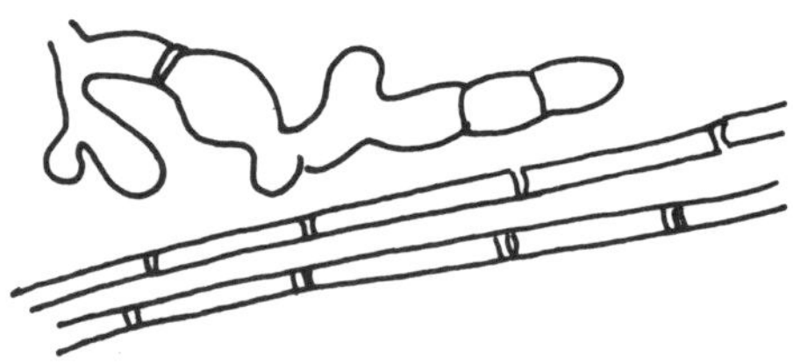

Thallus yellow to rust colored, heaped up or cerebriforme; or white and somewhat flat, with yellow to rust colored, glabrous concentric zones. Hyphae irregular, fragmented, and swollen, or else thick and straight with prominent double septa (suggesting bamboo). May mutate to peach tan forms suggestive of M. audouinii, 19 M. ferrugineum (CHP), fluorescent tinea capitis, principally East Asia, North and tropical Africa, Eastern Europe (also check 13 M. canis, 56 T. soudanense, and 16 M. audouinii).

58 Thallus usually heaped or spreading with radial "alluvial" folds. Color of thallus lemon yellow to ochraceous - Plate II(47). Stimulated by thiamine to produce a flatter more downy thallus, sometimes with tear-shaped microaleuriospores. Usually connected with inflammatory ringworm and large spore ectothrix hair parasitism. . . 47 <u>T. verrucosum</u> (ochraceum form) (RHP to CHP), cattle, principally tinea corporis, tinea capitis, and tinea barbae (also check 59 T. schoenleinii, 40 T. mentagrophytes, 19 M. ferrugineum, and 13 M. canis).

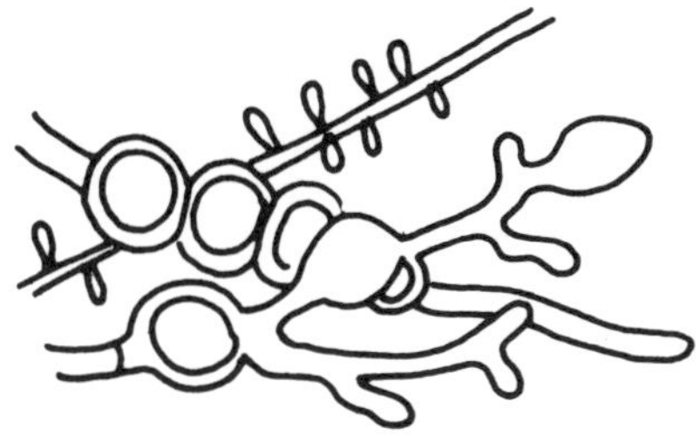

Thallus usually heaped and much convoluted or warty. Color of thallus orange to honey-colored or brown, not bright yellow - Plate III(61, 59). Growth may be stimulated by thiamine but aleuriospores not produced. Associated with tokelau, a tropical form of tinea corporis restricted to South Asia, South Pacific Islands, and endemic areas in central and south America; or with favus, a form of tinea capitis, world-wide, but principally in East Europe, USSR, North Africa, Middle East, Iceland. Locally endemic elsewhere. 63

59 Thallus brown or honey colored. 60

Thallus white or near white. 61

60 Thallus initially cream white, with a heaped glabrous surface, usually becoming more or less chocolate brown with maturity and producing brown diffusing pigment - Plate III(58). Microaleuriospores may be present. . . 58 <u>T. yaoundei</u> (CHP), principally tinea capitis, endemic equatorial Africa (also check 55 T. gourvilii and 54 T. violaceum).

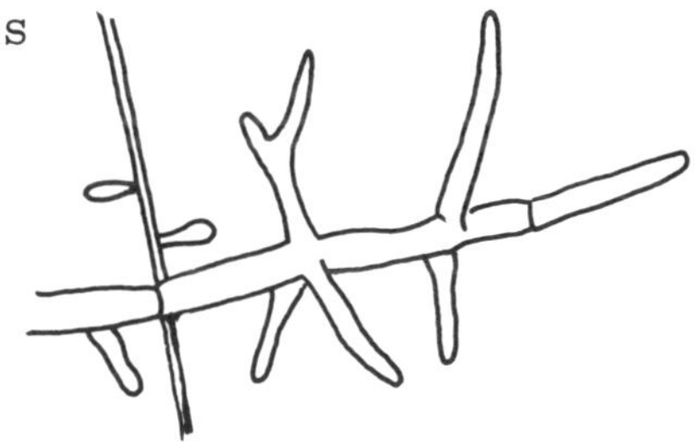

Thallus honey colored to brown with a cerebriform or verrucose, glabrous surface, not becoming chocolate brown with maturity and not producing diffusing brown pigment - Plate III(47). Mycelia usually much branched with clubbed and antler-like tips. 61

61 Thallus heaped up or flat, white or grey, glabrous button-like and tough, or somewhat fuzzy or downy. With addition of thiamine becoming more or less flat and downy, sometimes with production of aleuriospores. Mycelia irregular, branched, antler-like, and clubbed. Growth and chlamydospore production enhanced at 37°C. (If antler-like, clubbed hyphae and chlamydospores are not a conspicuous feature check T. violaceum var. glabrum). Associated with inflammatory ringworm and large spore ectothrix hair parasitism. . . 47 <u>T. verrucosum</u> (RHP to CHP), cattle (also check 59 T. schoenleinii, 61 T. concentricum, 54 T. violaceum, and 50 T. rubrum).

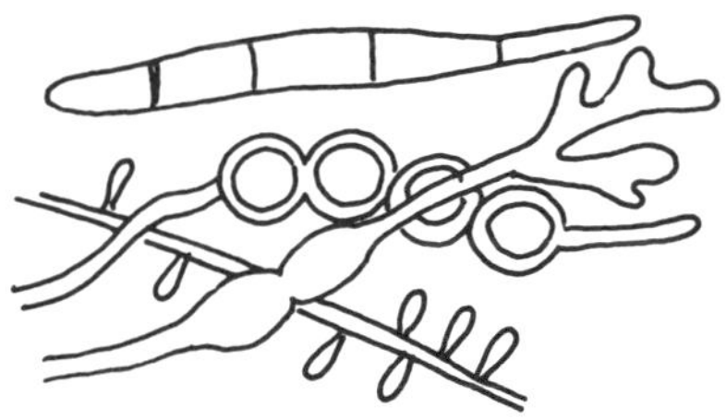

Thallus more or less cerebriform or folded and spreading, glabrous or somewhat fuzzy or downy, white to grey white or cream colored. Not producing aleuriospores with addition of thiamine. Hyphal elements frequently antler-like, or pectinate, or enlarged terminally. Associated with tinea imbricata, tinea corporis, favus type of tinea capitis, or fluorescent ectothrix tinea capitis.................................... **62**

62 Thallus grey to white, glabrous to fluffy, rapidly growing, and relatively friable. With addition of yeast extract, becoming more fluffy and radially folded. Mycelia with terminal inflated and bulbous hyphal elements and pectinate hyphae. Macro-aleuriospores of the M. audouinii type sometimes present. . . 16 <u>M. audouinii var. rivalieri</u> (CHP), principally fluorescent ectothrix tinea capitis (also check 59 T. schoenleinii).

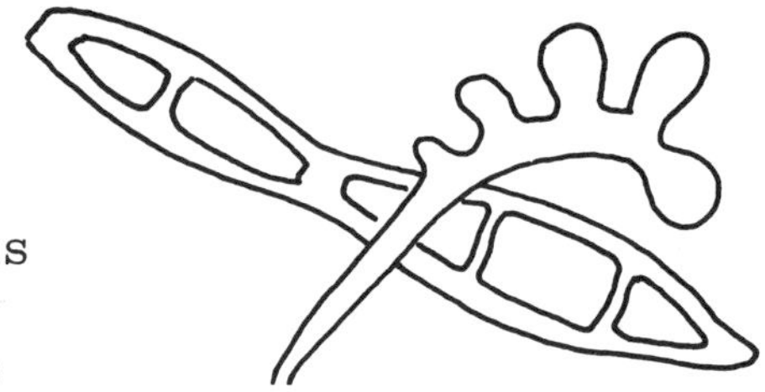

Thallus usually tough and leathery, not frankly fluffy, on first isolation entirely glabrous, and not exhibiting a marked change of morphology with addition of yeast extract... **63**

63 Thallus in subculture often becoming grey white and somewhat spreading with radial folds and tending to crack the agar. Branched antler and nail head hyphae present. Not stimulated by thiamine. . 59 <u>T. schoenleinii</u> (CHP), favus, principally tinea capitis. World-wide but principally North Africa, Eastern Europe, Russia, Middle East, and Iceland (also check 47 T. verrucosum, 61 T. concentricum, 19 M. ferrugineum and 54 T. violaceum).

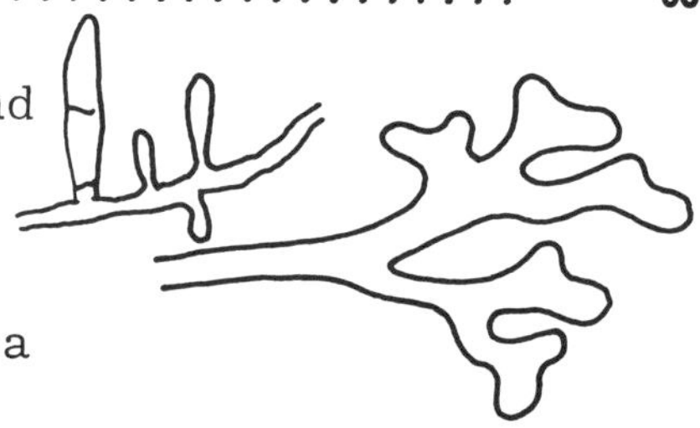

Thallus not normally becoming grey white and spreading with radial folds if subcultured regularly. Thallus predominantly heaped and cerebriforme. Branched hyphae frequent, nail head hyphae not well developed. . . 61 <u>T. concentricum</u> (CHP), tokelau, tinea corporis only, tropical and restricted to South Pacific area, South Asia, and limited foci in Central and South America (also check 47 T. verrucosum, 59 T. schoenleinii, and 50 T. rubrum).

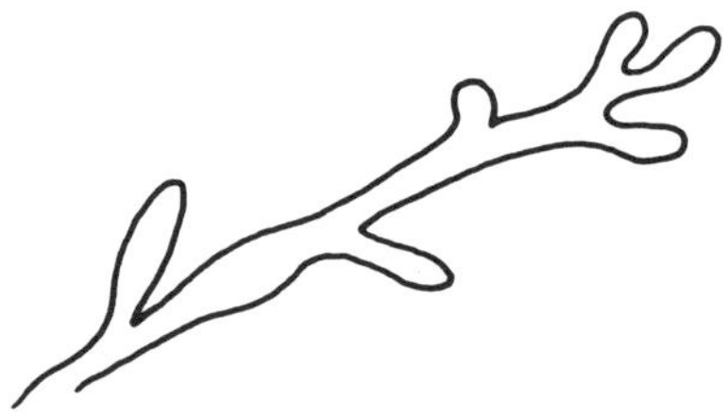

64 Culture producing abundant rectangular arthrospores (Arthroaleuriospores) and few or no micro- or macroaleuriospores. . . 50 <u>T. rubrum</u> (CHP), 36 <u>T. gloriae</u> (NHP), 40 <u>T. mentagrophytes</u> (CHP), 13 <u>M. canis</u> (CHP), 73 <u>Malbranchea sp.</u> (NHP), etc. Differential separation based upon evidence of microscopic and macroscopic morphology otherwise typical of these species.

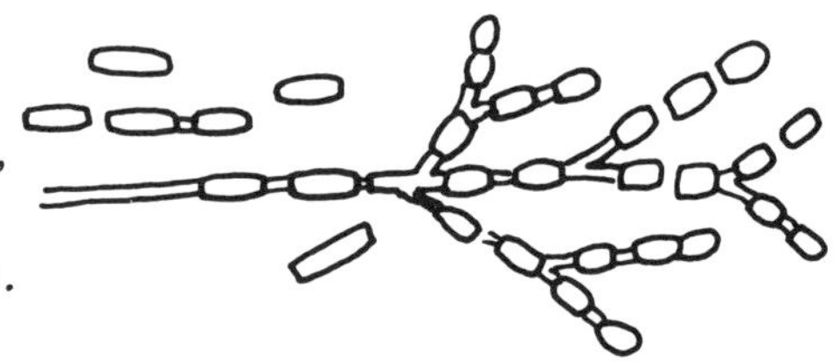

Culture not producing abundant rectangular arthrospores or aleuriospores as a predominant or only microscopic feature........................ **65**

65 Margin of growing thallus yellow beneath or thallus predominantly yellow beneath. 66

Undersurface of growing thallus not yellow, predominantly or at the growing margin. 69

66 Surface of thallus powdery, white to cream, flat, remaining friable and powdery when mature - Plate II(44). Undersurface with clear yellow diffusing pigment. Microaleuriospores usually uniform, narrow, club-shaped, abundant, and in effect clustered on terminal hyphal branches. Macroaleuriospores frequently present and club-shaped, usually variable in size, the smallest intergrading with microaleuriospores. 44 T. erinacei (RHP), carried by hedgehog (also check 40 T. mentagrophytes and 45 T. equinum).

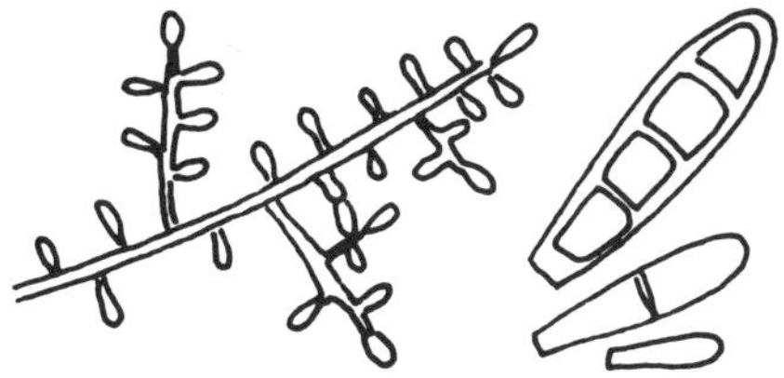

Mature thallus fluffy, or folded and suede-like, and forming skin-like pellicle on the agar rather than powdery and friable - Plates I(13), II(45), and IV(40). 67

67 Surface of mature thallus frequently with loose cottony tufts and sometimes sparse glabrous areas, and flat and somewhat coarse and spreading, usually with 10 or more radial grooves. Microaleuriospores usually few and slender club-shaped or teardrop-shaped. Further study of culture usually reveals large, spindle-shaped macroaleuriospores (see item 4). . . .13 M. canis (CHP) cat (also check 19 M. ferrugineum and 16 M. audouinii).

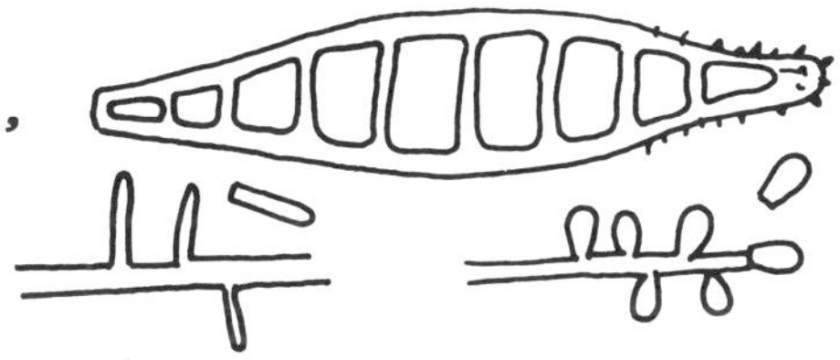

Surface of mature thallus densely and usually uniformly downy, velvety, or suede-like, flat or folded, and white, grey, tan, or pink. 68

68 Microaleuriospores usually predominantly lateral on non-terminal hyphae and variously spherical, teardrop-shaped, or club-shaped, sometimes with slender attenuated bases or stalks. Surface of thallus white to brownish or pink, fluffy or velvety, usually forming a compact folded pellicle on the agar. Undersurface of thallus usually yellow or yellow at the margin, becoming reddish or brownish centrally. Macroaleuriospores club-shaped, but usually rare on Sabouraud Agar and associated with microaleuriospores clustered on terminal hyphal branches. . .45 T. equinum (RHP), horse. Some isolates may be confirmed by demonstrating a requirement for nicotinic acid (also check 40 T. mentagrophytes var. quinkeanum, 44 T. erinacei, 13 M. canis, 52 T. tonsurans var sulfureum, 50 T. rubrum, and 38 T. simii).

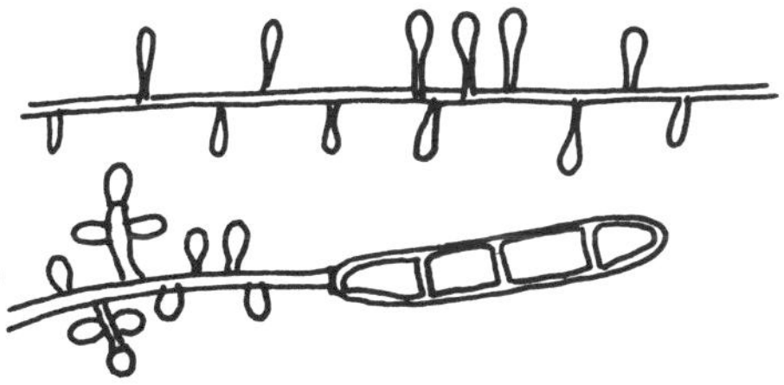

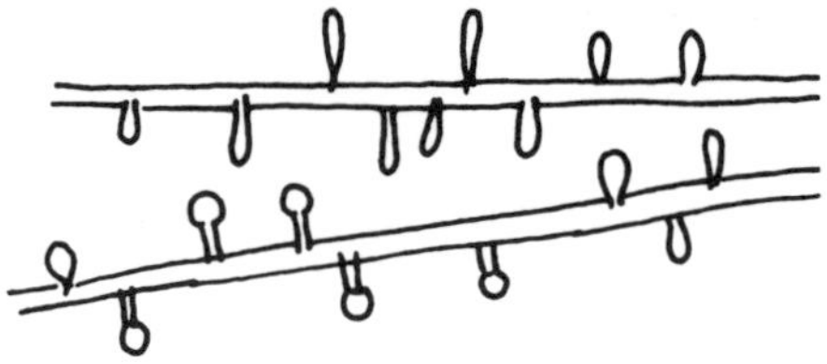

Lateral microaleuriospores spherical, egg-shaped, teardrop-shaped, peg-shaped, or club-shaped, but usually not conspicuously on slender stalks, or stalks if present consisting of a short supporting pillar of about the same diameter as the microaleuriospores. . .
40 T. mentagrophytes (var. quinkeanum) (RHP) rodents,
T. mentagrophytes var nodulare (CHP) principally tinea pedis (also check 50 T. rubrum, 36 T. gloriae, and 52 T. tonsurans).

69 Undersurface of thallus developing a dark red or garnet red pigment, surface glabrous to fluffy, pink to white, or greenish - Plate II(49); III(50, 55): IV(50). 70

Undersurface of thallus not becoming distinctly red (may be brown, pinkish tan, or colorless) - Plates I(16); II(40); III(50, 52); IV(40). 72

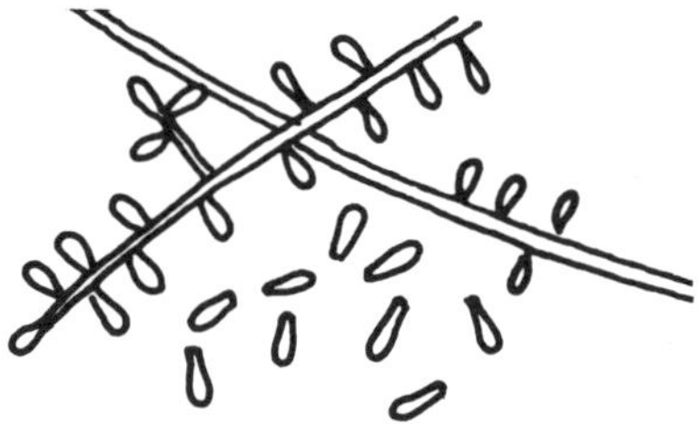

70 Surface of thallus more or less fluffy and white, pink or greenish. Mature thallus usually developing a venous blood undercolor as it matures (or on potato dextrose agar). Microaleuriospores usually small and peg-shaped and rare to exceedingly abundant. Macroaleuriospores, if present narrow, appearing long cylindrical. . .50 T. rubrum (CHP) principally tinea corporis, tinea pedis, and tinea manus (also check 49 T. megninii, 55 T. gourvilii, and 40 T. mentagrophytes var quinkeanum).

Surface and undersurface of thallus pink to garnet red, surface waxy, glabrous, fluffy, or suede-like. Microaleuriospores club-shaped or teardrop-shaped, rare to numerous but not exceedingly abundant. 71

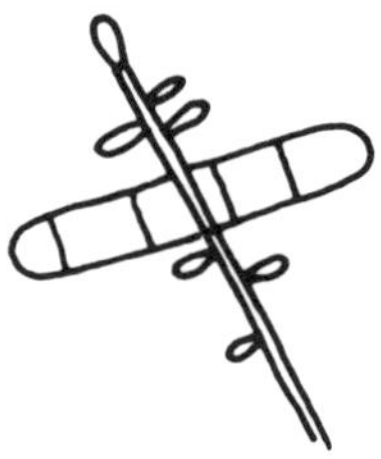

71 Thallus usually glabrous or waxy initially, and heaped and purplish pink to garnet red. Dark brown pigment may be produced beneath the thallus. Microaleuriospores usually few. . .55
T. gourvilii (CHP) principally endothrix tinea capitis. Tropical West Africa (also check 54 T. violaceum, 56 T. soudanense, 49 T. megninii, and T. yaoundei).

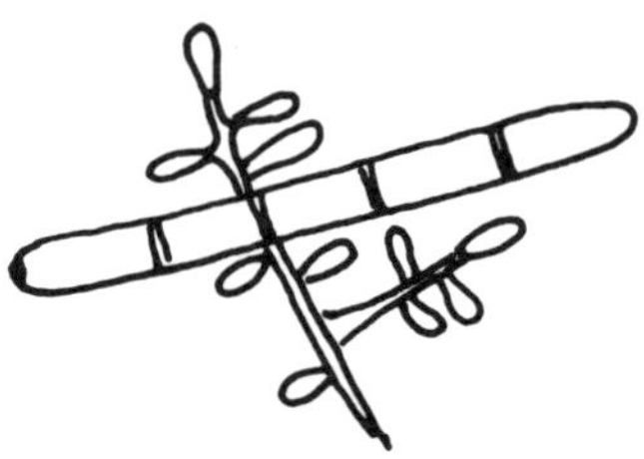

Thallus pink and downy or suede-like with radial furrows. Undersurface garnet red. Microaleurio-spores club-shaped to teardrop-shaped. Macro-aleuriospores narrow, appearing long cylindrical. Histidine requiring . .49 T. megninii (CHP) geographically restricted to Europe and Africa (need to distinguish from 40 T. rubrum by requirement for histidine) (also check 69 T. fluviomuniense and 55 T. gourvilii).

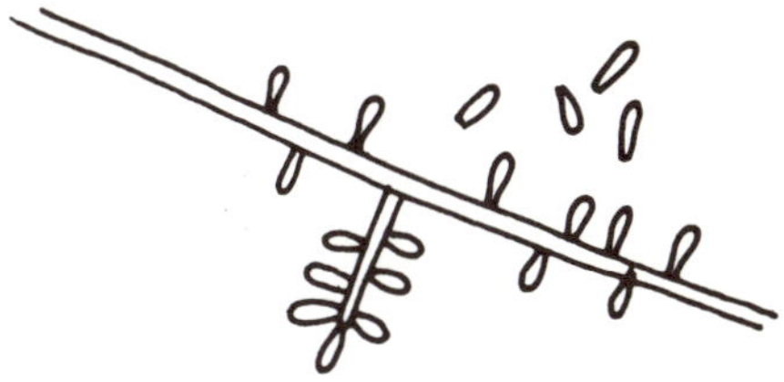

72 Thallus essentially white and fluffy, but producing a diffusing dark brown pigment- Plate III(50). aleuriospores lateral and peg-shaped . . . 50 T. rubrum (CHP), principally tinea corporis, tinea pedis, and tinea manus (also check 45 T. equinum).

Thallus not producing a diffusing brown pigment or brown surface. 73

73 Undersurface of thallus tinted with salmon or peach-tan or brown. 74

Undersurface of thallus colorless. 75

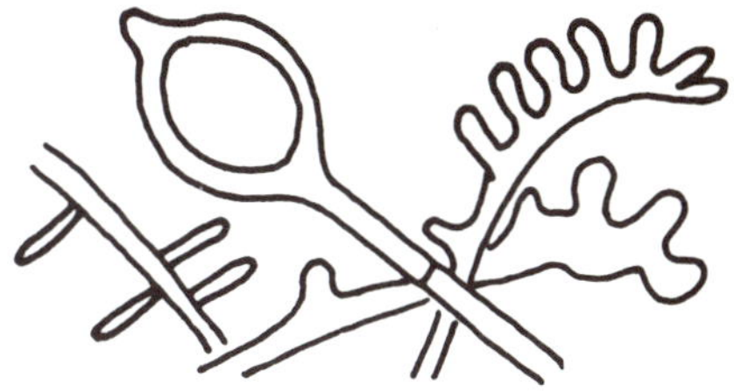

74 Surface of thallus flat and spreading, sparsely to densely and fluffy, developing radial furrows, and white, tan, or light pinkish brown. Microaleuriospores usually rare and pyriform to slender clavate. Macroaleuriospores usually absent. Terminal chlamydospores often present. Pectinate hyphae frequently present. . . 16 M. audouinii (CHP), principally tinea capitis (also check 52 T. tonsurans and 40 T. mentagrophytes).

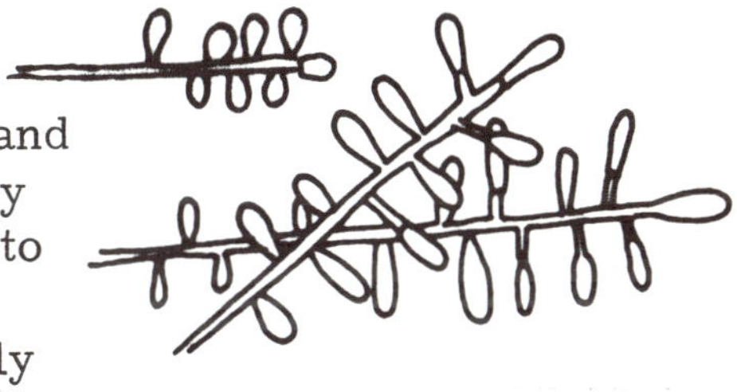

Surface of thallus somewhat powdery, white, yellow, or greyish, flat or becoming suede-like and folded with maturity. Microaleuriospores usually abundant and variable in size and shape, clavate to filiform. Terminal chlamydospores frequently present. . . 52 T. tonsurans (CHP), principally tinea capitis (also check 16 M. audouinii, 40 T. mentagrophytes and 50 T. rubrum).

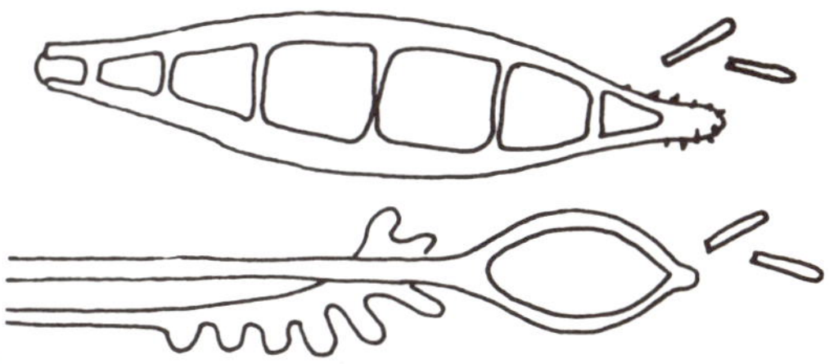

75 Thallus essentially colorless on surface and below, flat spreading usually developing radial grooves Advancing mycelium usually relatively coarse, straight, and succulent. Microaleuriospores pear-shaped to slender clavate and usually rare or absent. . . 13 M. canis (CHP), or 16 M. audouinii (CHP). Principally fluorescent tinea capits. Differentiate on rice media and by search for macroaleuriospores, pectinate hyphae, and terminal chlamydospores (also check 50 T. rubrum and 40 T. mentagrophytes).

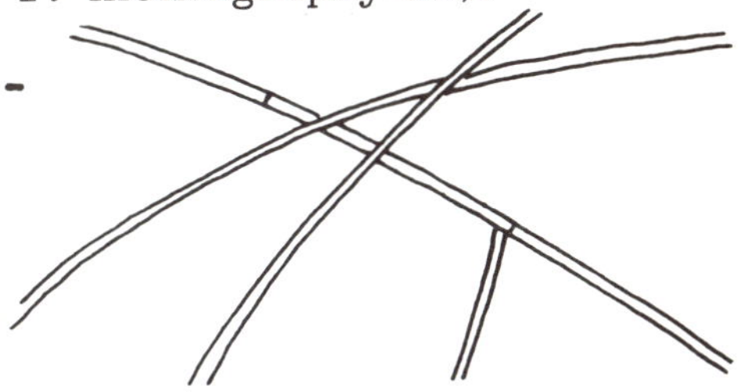

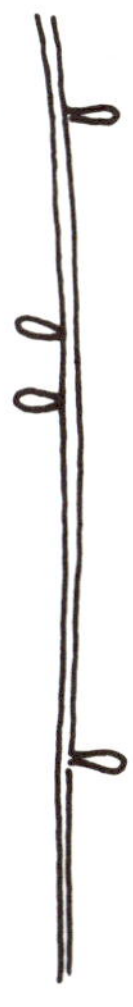

Thallus white, flat and more or less fluffy. Advancing mycelium usually thin and flexuous. Lateral, pear-shaped microaleuriospores rare or more or less common throughout the thallus. . . 50 T. rubrum (CHP), 40 T. mentagrophytes (CHP), and pleomorphic forms of other dermatophytes. Differentiate T. rubrum from T. mentagrophytes by hair perforation and urease tests. These are difficult and often insolvable problems of identification. If the thallus is fluffy and no macro- or microaleuriospores or other special microscopic features are present, the culture is probably unidentifiable, constituting a completely pleomorphic dermatophyte or other fungus classed taxonomically as "Mycelia Sterilia".

Dermatophyte Test Medium (DTM)

Used for isolating dermatophytes. This is a selective medium which excludes most bacteria and many contaminant fungi, combined with a yellow → red pH indicator which is quickly affected by dermatophytes and related fungi to permit their early recognition. In our opinion DTM replaces other media for the isolation of dermatophytes. Where identification of species is not required in order to institute treatment, positive growth and color change on DTM may be relied upon to have 98 percent accuracy in diagnosis of dermatophyte infections in man. Data is not yet available to assess the reliability of DTM as a simplified diagnostic procedure in veterinary medicine. (Taplin, D. Zaias, N., Rebell, G., and Blank, H., 1969. Arch. Derm. 99:203-209).

Warning: Substitution of ingredients from sources other than those indicated may change the characteristics and selectivity of the medium.

Distilled water, 1000 ml
Phytone (BBL), 10 gm
Dextrose, 10 gm
Agar Agar (BBL or Difco), 20 gm
Phenol Red Solution, 40 ml
0.8 N HCl, 6 ml
Cycloheximide (Actidione, Upjohn), 0.5 gm
Gentamicin sulfate, 0.1 gm of active drug = 100 μg/ml
Chlortetracycline HCl, 0.1 gm = 100 μg/ml

1) Add phytone, dextrose, and agar to 1000 ml distilled water and boil to dissolve agar.

2) Add 40 ml of phenol red solution while stirring. (Phenol red solution: 0.5 gm Difco Bacto-Phenol Red dissolved in 15 ml 0.1 N NaOH made up to 100 ml with distilled water).

3) Add 6 ml 0.8 N HCl added while stirring.

4) Dissolve 0.5 gm cycloheximide in 2 ml acetone and add to hot medium while stirring.

5) Dissolve sufficient gentamicin sulfate powder (Schering Corp., New Jersey) in 2 ml distilled water to give a final concentration in the medium of 100 μg/ml of active drug. The amount is dependent on the assay of each sample of gentamicin. A sample with activity of 500 μg/mgm would, for example, require 0.2 gm to be added to each liter of medium.

6) Autoclave at 12 lbs for 10 minutes and cool to approximately 47°C.

7) Dissolve 0.1 gm chlortetracycline HCl (American Cyanamid, New York) in 25 ml sterile distilled water and add to medium while stirring.

8) Pour plates or dispense in 1 ounce wide mouthed bottles (8 ml per bottle and cool on the slant).

9) Store under refrigeration for maximum shelf life.

10) After inoculation leave caps loose to allow adequate growth and development of indicator color change. Optimum temperature for incubation is 28° C to 30°C. Excessively cool room temperature may delay growth.

11) Color change of indicator should be interpreted not later than two weeks after inoculation. Longer incubation may produce false positive results from slow growing contaminant fungi and does not increase the recovery of dermatophytes.

(see also reference page 116)

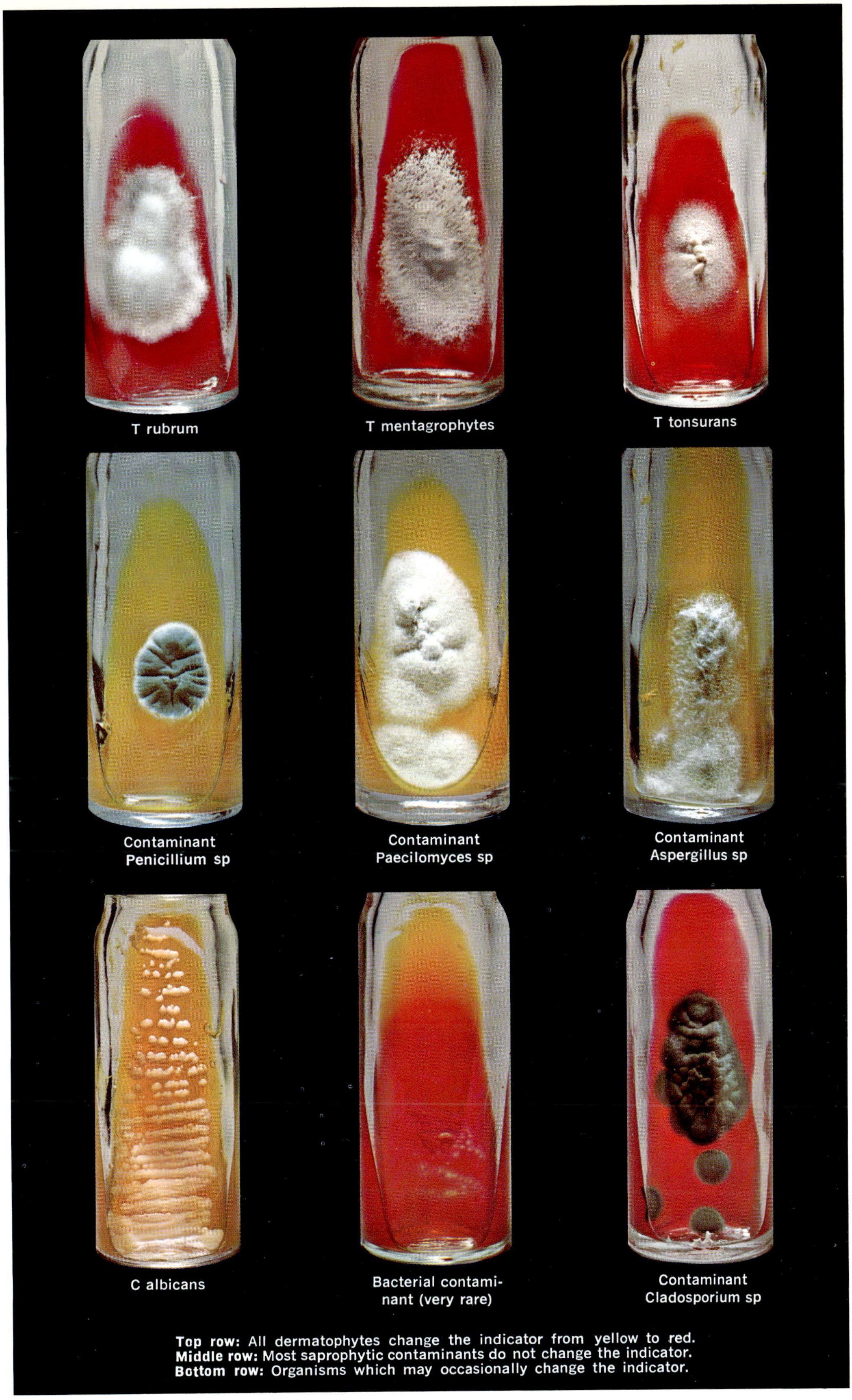

Top row: All dermatophytes change the indicator from yellow to red.
Middle row: Most saprophytic contaminants do not change the indicator.
Bottom row: Organisms which may occasionally change the indicator.

Reprinted from the Archives of Dermatology
February 1969, Volume 99

Sabouraud's Agar (Dextrose Peptone Agar)

Used for routine cultivation of dermatophytes.

Distilled water	1000 ml	Dextrose	40 gm
Peptone*	10 gm	Agar Agar	20 gm

Bring to boil to dissolve agar agar and autoclave (120°C, 15 minutes). If commercial dehydrated prepared medium is used, add 5 gm agar agar per liter. Sabouraud's agar is used at pH 5.6.

* Several peptones are used (Difco neopeptone, BBL phytone, Oxoid mycological peptone, etc.). The color plates in this manual show cultures on Difco dehydrated Sabouraud's Dextrose Agar which contains neopeptone.

Modifications of Sabouraud's Agar

1) Addition of yeast extract (5 gms per liter). More closely approximates the medium used by Sabouraud to identify dermatophytes - growth and morphology are enhanced.

2) Without dextrose. Sabouraud's "conservation" agar - used for maintaining stock cultures. Also for differentiating M. persicolor from T. mentagrophytes.

3) With Chloramphenicol and Cycloheximide. A selective isolation medium (now supplanted by DTM). With DTM, the yield of dermatophytes is greater due principally to the more effective bacteriostasis. To add chloramphenicol: suspend 50 mg in 10 ml 95 percent ethanol, add this to one liter of the boiling medium and quickly cool. Autoclave chloramphenicol medium at 118°C for 10 minutes only. For cycloheximide addition see DTM.

Some cultures in color plates I and IV are shown on chloramphenicol-cycloheximide medium (Mycosel, BBL). Growth features are close to those obtained on DTM.

4) Dilute Sabouraud's Agar. Used recently in demonstrating macroaleuriospores of M. ferrugineum. The dilution effect can be obtained by transfering a block of Sabouraud's Agar culture to the surface of 2 percent agar agar in water (or in water containing 0.1 gm KH_2PO_4 and 0.1 gm $MgSO_4$ 7 H_2O per liter). Macroaleuriospores were observed as the thallus grew out into the nutrient free medium.

Potato Dextrose Agar

Used for maintaining stock cultures of geophilic dermatophytes; and to distinguish M. audouinii from M. canis and T. rubrum from T. mentagrophytes.

Potatoes 250 gms (peel, slice, boil in 100 ml dist. water, filter and add the following to the filtrate):

Dextrose	20 gms	
Agar Agar	20 gms	Distilled water to make 1 liter final volume

Bring to a boil to dissolve the agar agar and autoclave (120°C, 10 minutes). Commercial dehydrated potato dextrose agar tends to be of uneven quality.

Freezing Agar

(Kuehn, Orr, and Ghosh, 1961. Mycopath. Mycol. Appl. 14:215-229)

Used to maintain stock cultures of geophilic dermatophytes in deep freeze. Used recently in demonstrating macroaleuriospores of M. ferrugineum.

Potatoes 200 gms (without peeling, slice, autoclave in 500 ml water at 120°C, 15 minutes, mash and filter through gauze. Add the following to the filtrate):

Agar Agar	20 gm		
Dextrose	8 gm	Activated Charcoal (carbon)	0.5 gm
Yeast Extract	1 gm	Distilled water to make one liter final volume	

Bring to boil to dissolve the agar agar and autoclave (120°C, 15 minutes). To use as a stock culture medium, inoculate and permit the fungus to grow. After growth has progressed enough to obtain mature sporulation in the central portion of the thallus, put culture in deep freeze. Subculture directly from frozen state

Dieldrin Media

Mycologic media can be made lethal to fungus mites without affecting fungi by adding 20 parts per million of dieldrin (personal communication F. J. Roth, Jr., University of Miami).

Dieldrin*	200 mg
Acetone	10 ml

Add 1 ml of dieldrin solution per liter of media before or after autoclaving.

* Dieldrin is a poisonous pesticide. Handle cautiously, avoid contaminating skin, and do not pipette by mouth. Velsicol Chemical Corp., 341 East Ohio Street, Chicago, Illinois 60611.

Rice Grain Medium

Used to distinguish M. audouinii from M. canis and M. distortum.

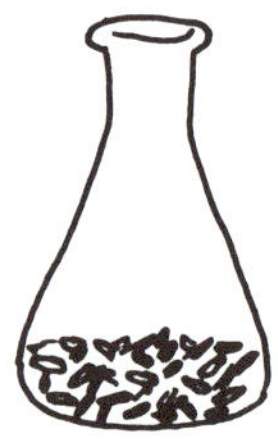

Polished white rice (without added vitamins)	8 gm
Distilled water	25 mls

Place these quantities in individual 125 ml erlenmeyer flasks or large tubes, autoclave (120°C, 15 minutes). Inoculate with small fragments of growing culture.

Media to Test for Vitamin, Amino Acid, and Nitrogen Requirements

Nicotinic acid (niacin), see page 46; thiamine, see page 48; inositol, see page 48; histidine, see page 49; growth on NH_4NO_3 and histidine, see page 49.

Urease Test

(Philpot, C., 1967. Sabouraudia 5:189-193)

Used to differentiate T. rubrum from T. erinacei from T. mentagrophytes. For T. rubrum use in combination with hair perforation test and growth on Potato Dextrose Agar. Also possibly useful in separating M. ferrugineum (slight urease activity) from T. soudanense (no urease activity).

Peptone (mycological, Oxoid)	1 gm	Glucose	5 gm
NaCl	5 gm	Agar Agar	20 gm
KH_2PO_4	2 gm	Distilled water	1000 ml

Add 6 ml phenol red solution (0.2% in 50% ethanol). Autoclave (115°C, 15 min). Cool to 50°C, add 100 ml of filter sterilized 20% aqueous solution of urea. Slant in tubes or pour plates. Inoculate with small bits of culture to be tested. Urease activity causes an alkaline (yellow→red) pH change. (Since all dermatophytes produce an alkaline pH change with growth, only early pH changes in urea-rich medium are indicative of urease activity).

T. rubrum	T. mentagrophytes	T. erinacei
Urease activity weak or absent (no pH change before 14 days) * granular types may have weak urease activity. (pH change in 7 - 14 days).	(+) mating types; strong urease activity (pH change before 7 days) (-) mating types; weak urease activity (pH change in 7 - 10 days) (Padhye, A., 1970. Bact. Proc., p. 120).	No urease activity

In Vitro Perforation of Hair

(Ajello, L. and Georg, L.K., 1957. Mycopath. Mycol. Appl. 8:3-17)

Although there have been reports of hair perforation by T. rubrum, the test appears to differentiate most or all strains from T. mentagrophytes if performed as follows:

Place short (1 cm) strand of prepubertal human hair in petri dishes and sterilize by autoclaving (120°C for 10 minutes). Add 25 ml sterile distilled water and 2 to 3 drops of sterile 10% yeast extract. Inoculate plates with small fragments of test fungus culture grown on Sabouraud's agar. Examine for perforations at intervals up to 4 weeks by removing single hairs from the plates and scanning them under the microscope in a drop of lacto-phenol cotton blue, slightly warmed, under a coverslip. Examination with KOH permits visualization of the perforating organ (English, M.P., 1968. Sabouraudia 6:218-227), see page 5.

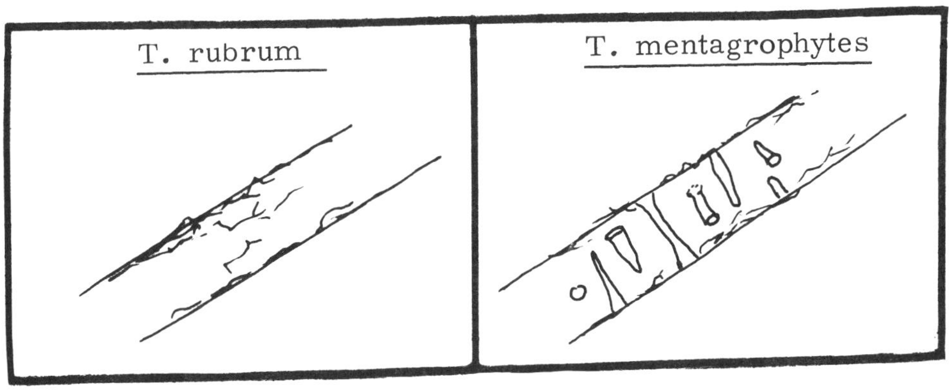

Lacto-Phenol Cotton Blue Mounting Fluid

Used as a fluid mount between slide and coverslip for examining transparent tape mounts and other preparations of fungus hyphae for microscopic observation. The stain is not readily water-miscible.

Phenol	20 gm (melt in warm water, then weigh)
Lactic Acid	20 gm
Glycerin	40 gm
Cotton Blue (Poirrier's Blue)	0.05 gm
Distilled water	20 ml

Add in order: 1) lactic acid and glycerin and distilled water, 2) add phenol and dissolve with even heat, 3) add cotton blue and dissolve, 4) filter through paper.

Diluted Albert's Solution I (Mounting Fluid)

This stain is used as a wet mount for fragments of aerial growth (scraped off the surface of the thallus with a needle). It gives crisp details of the walls and compartments of macroaleuriospores (see figures 1 - 21, Plate V). Water-miscible and not suitable for tape mounts.

Toluidin Blue	0.15 gm	95 percent Ethanol	2 ml
Malachite Green	0.2 gm	Distilled water	110 ml
Glacial acetic acid	1 ml		

For use, dilute stock solution (above) 1:2 with distilled water and add 10 percent glycerine (30 ml glycerine for 300 ml stain).

KOH (Mounting Fluid)

Used to search for fungus in skin scrapings and hair. Twenty percent KOH causes the keratin cells to swell and clear, and provides an advantageous refractive index to reveal the fungus hyphae.

With DMSO		Without DMSO	
Distilled water	60 ml	Distilled water	80 ml
Potassium hydroxide (KOH)	20 gms	Potassium hydroxide (KOH)	20 gms
Dimethyl Sulfoxide (DMSO)	40 ml	Glycerine	20 ml

If used without DMSO, the slide must be slightly warmed to promote clearing. Addition of DMSO permits quick examination often without warming. Addition of DMSO or glycerine prevents rapid drying of the fluid, permits observation of the slide for up to 24 or 48 hours. Slides may be ringed with fingernail polish to save for longer periods. To provide a semi-permanent preparation, the KOH must be replaced by glycerine by cappillary displacement. Blot at one side of slide and slowly add glycerine from the other side.

CLINICAL METHODS

General Advice

Two keys to successful laboratory diagnosis of dermatophyte infections are: first, selective culture from scales, nail material, and hairs observed to be KOH positive, and second, a specimen of scales, nail or hair free from extraneous material such as dirt, sebum , ointments, antifungal agents, cosmetics, and so on. The lesion may be washed with soap and water. Also, large pieces of scale, callous, nail, or tufts of hair implanted in the agar have a poor chance of success. Bacteria present and other factors tend to kill the fungus and prevent its outgrowth from the specimen. Depending on the inflammatory tissue reaction and other factors the hyphae and arthrospores of dermatophyte fungi can be very abundant or very rare in the lesion. It is usually desirable and often necessary to make several cultures, especially from lesions which are chronic or which are highly inflammatory, or which have been treated. Repeated KOH examinations may be required to demonstrate the fungus. Well chosen scales, fairly deep and traumatic scrapings from active parts of the lesion, vesicle tops, and selected hairs are the best material to examine and culture. The material selected for culture should be pressed into the surface of the agar to ensure good contact with the medium but not buried in it.

Making a KOH Mount

A sample is placed on the slide, a drop of KOH added, and a coverslip pressed down on it (or else the specimen is first picked up on a plastic coverslip utilizing the electrostatic charge, see below). The slide is then warmed slightly to hasten dissolution of the keratinized cells by the KOH. If DMSO is used in the KOH, warming may not be necessary. If glycerine is used in the KOH, the slide may be stored for later examination.

Use of Plastic Coverslip*

These are handy for two reasons:
1) they can be pressed down on uneven or gritty matter without breaking, and
2) they have a surface charge which causes epidermal scales, nail particles, and hair stubs to adhere to them. The fine epidermal scrapings can be picked up in abundance by the coverslip as indicated in figure 1 and then the coverslip placed over a drop of KOH on a slide for examination.

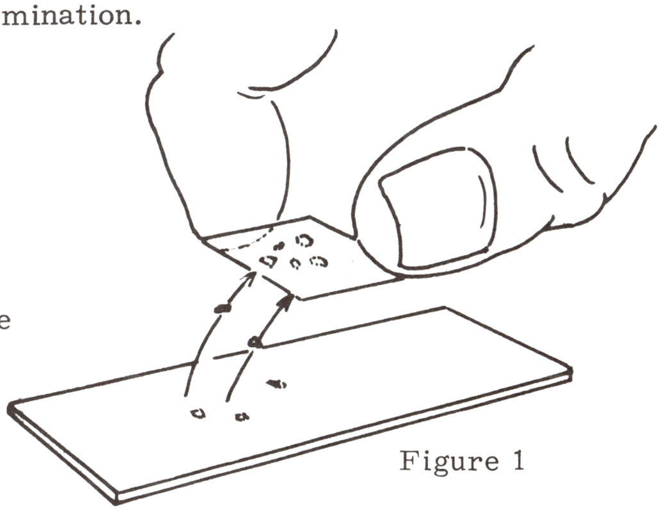

Figure 1

DTM Touch Plate Method for Culturing Tinea Capitis

A petri dish of DTM is pressed firmly against the scalp lesion, picking up spores from the infected hairs. The plate is then incubated at 30-34°C. In our experience this is the most rapid and satisfactory technique for culturing tinea capitis caused by the fluorescent Microsporum and endothrix Trichophyton species. It is especially useful in school epidemics. Many isolates are usually obtained on the surface of the agar at the site of contact with the lesion.

* diSPo Slips, Scientific Products

(See reference bottom of page 116)

Clinical Methods - Cont.

To Select Parasitized Hairs for Microscopic Examination or Culture

In endothrix human infections it is often necessary to pick the coiled hair ("black dots") from the scalp with a scalpel as shown in Figure 2. In ectothrix infections (or in favus) hair stubs may usually be plucked with forceps as shown in Figure 3. In both types of infections however, one may simply scrape the scalp lesion with a scalpel and catch the hair fragments and scales on a slide or other surface from which they can be picked up with a plastic coverslip.

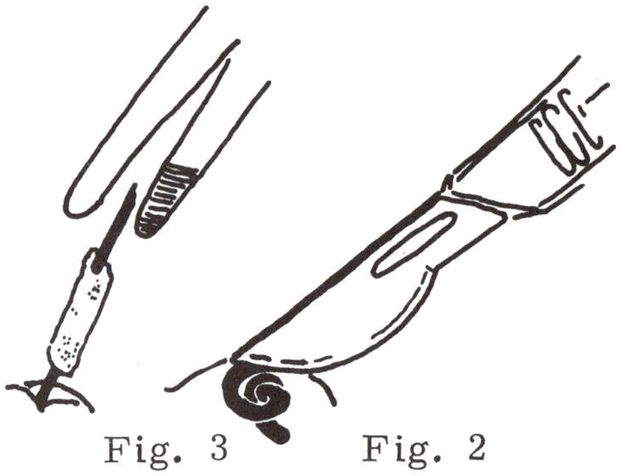

Fig. 3 Fig. 2

Ultraviolet (Wood's Light) Examination for Fluorescent Hairs

Hairs infected with the parasitic Microsporum species may be detected by the yellow-green fluorescence in 3660 A ultraviolet light. The skin itself does not fluoresce. In veterinary medicine the Wood's light is useful to detect M. canis infections in cats, dogs, and other small animals. Although low output Wood's lights or "mineral lights" are often used, they are not dependable when hair fluorescence is not intense. The 100 watt Blak-Ray lamp, or a lamp of comparable output is recommended.

To Culture Highly Inflammatory Lesions of the Body, Beard, and Scalp (Kerion)

These are sometimes difficult to culture because the fungus and parasitized hairs may be scarce and may be in pus in the depths of the follicles or small abcesses in a granulomatous tissue reaction. Plucking and culturing hairs and also pus on DTM is recommended. Sparse chains of spores may be found in the hairs by KOH examination. The Gram stain often reveals bits of hyphae in pus more successfully than a KOH preparation. Tinea corporis and tinea barbae of this type is frequently associated with T. mentagrophytes, T. verrucosum, and sometimes with T. rubrum.

Examination of Toe Interspaces, Groins, and Other Intertrigenous Sites

The failure to culture dermatophytes from KOH positive scales is sometimes due to misidentification of filamentous forms of Candida albicans as dermatophyte hyphae in the KOH preparation. A Gram stain of intertriginous lesions will usually reveal the difference, since the C. albicans takes an intense, solid Gram stain, and in association with the hyphal yeasts cells are seen which may be overlooked in the KOH preparation. The admonition to make cultures selectively from material demonstrated to be KOH positive is particularly important in the case of intertriginous lesions, since the growing fungus may be confined to certain active places or borders of the lesion, and be rare or absent in other places which may yet show the signs and symptoms associated with dermatophytosis. Probably focal itching is a relatively reliable evidence of active fungus (or of C. albicans). Not infrequently several to many KOH preparations are required before the fungus is discovered.

Palms and Soles

Scaling lesions usually require persistence and repeated KOH preparations to discover the dermatophyte. Hyphae are frequently but not always found in the roof of plantar vesicles. Palmar vesicles usually have no fungus.

Culturing Nails

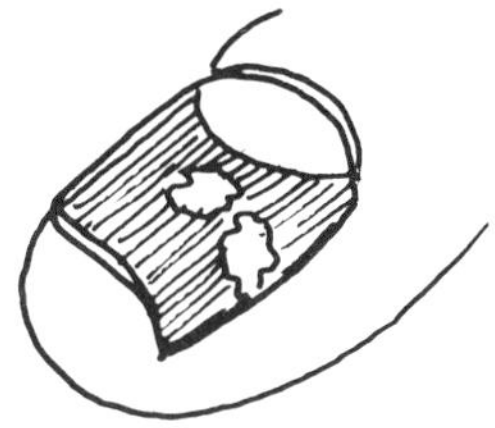

Fig. 5

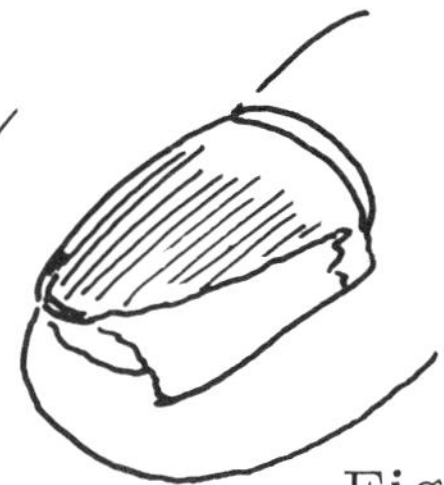

Fig. 4

Bacteria and other factors limit the chance of isolating a dermatophyte from large pieces of nail. There are two main types of nail infection. 1) The type invading beneath the nail plate and 2) the white spot type invading the top surface of the nail plate. In the deep type (fig. 4) KOH positive material (often crumbly) may be obtained from beneath the nail plate (or by whittling through it), and spread out on the agar. In the superficial white spot type of onychomycosis (fig. 5) (usually caused by T. mentagrophytes) the white chalky spots on the nail plate are easily scraped off and spread on agar. Non-dermatophyte fungi may be involved in nail infections, and a percentage of clinically suggestive nails seem to harbor no filamentous fungi at all. (Zaias, N., 1966. Superficial White Onychomycosis, Sabouraudia 5:99-103).

Culturing Animals for Ringworm Infections

There is more trouble with cycloheximide resistant fungus contaminants in cultures from animals. Before making the culture, the hair on the lesions should be first clipped and the sites thoroughly washed with soap and water. The culture should consist of clean scrapings of epidermal scales and the selective culture of broken or fluorescent hairs, rather than inoculation of the agar with matted and crusted tufts of hair from the lesions without prior cleansing. Multiple cultures are recommended whenever a contamination problem can be anticipated. The pH indicator in DTM is particularly advantageous in detecting the early outgrowth of dermatophytes among contaminant fungi. Isolation of T. verrucosum (cattle ringworm) is favored at 37°C.

Contaminant Fungi

The problem of distinguishing dermatophytes from other fungi is greatly simplified if DTM is used. Dermatophytes pathogenic for man or animals grow well on DTM and rapidly turn the pH indicator red. Many common contaminants of dermatophyte cultures fail to grow on DTM or do not change the indicator color. The non-dermatophytic fungi which most frequently grow on DTM include Cladosporium spp., Scopulariopsis brevicaulis, some strains of Penicillium spp., Aspergillus spp., and Cephalosporium spp., Geotrichum candidum and some isolates of Candida albicans. These are macroscopically and microscopically rather easily differentiated from dermatophytes (see plate opposite page 106). A special class of contaminants, however, consist of T. terrestre, Chrysosporium spp., and other Keratinophilic soil fungi which are related to the pathogenic dermatophytes. These fungi are described briefly on pages 70-72.

EXAMINATION, MAINTENANCE, STORAGE, AND SHIPMENT OF CULTURES

Microscopic Preparations from Cultures to Show Aleuriospores

These are easily made with transparent pressure-sensitive tape as devised by F. Roth, Jr., University of Miami. Use No. 800 acetate-backed tape, Minnesota Mining and Mfg. Company. A flag of tape is fastened to a wooden applicator stick (figure 6) and the sticky surface touched to the surface of the thallus just proximal to the advancing periphery. The tape is then pressed sticky side down on a slide with a drop of lacto-phenol cotton blue stain and examined under the microscope directly. The tape selectively removes branches of hyphae bearing conidia and avoids the taxonomically valueless vegetative mycelium.

Favic hyphae of T. schoenleinii are best seen in a fragment of colony cut out with wire knife, made by flattening the end of a paper clip with a hammer (figure 7). These preparations are teased slightly and pressed out under a plastic coverslip with a drop of lacto-phenol cotton blue.

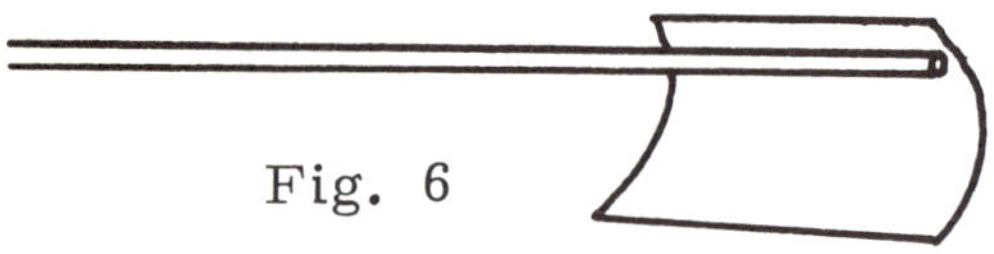

Fig. 6

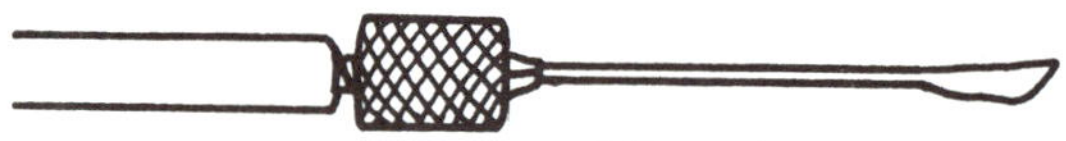

Fig. 7

Slide Cultures

Usually provide the best microscopic preparations for preservation and photography. Place a thin square of agar medium (containing gentamicin) on a sterile slide in a petri dish over blotting paper kept moist with sterile distilled water. The slide may be supported by a bent glass rod. Inoculate the edges of the agar block with the fungus culture and cover the block with a sterile coverslip. When the desired morphology has developed remove the coverslip with mycelia adhering to it and mount it on a fresh slide with a drop of lacto phenol cotton blue. The preparation may be sealed with fingernail polish. The agar blocks are cut out of thin-poured culture plates.

To Maintain Growing Laboratory Cultures for Study, Mutation (Pleomorphism)

The rapid mutational deterioration of fungi from the genetic state in which they are isolated from nature has in the case of dermatophytes been called "pleomorphism". These changes seem to be irreversible. Since they result from gene mutations or mitotic chromosome aberrations, it would seem possible to keep the original type by subculturing from the unmutated parts of the mycelium. Unfortunately pleomorphic mutants quickly overgrow the original thallus type. Repeated transfer of a culture from slant to slant inevitable results in a completely pleomorphic culture, with little trace of its original character. Streak out subcultures on an agar plate to isolate individual spores (using the technique employed to obtain single colonies in bacteriology). The original form can be re-isolated by subculturing typical thalli arising from single spores. In non-sporulating dermatophytes, streak out hyphal fragments or coarse homogenates. Potato dextrose agar, freezing agar, and Sabouraud's agar without dextrose (but with yeast extract) are better than Sabouraud's dextrose agar for storing growing cultures and will reduce the frequency of transfers required to control pleomorphism.

Control of Mycophagic Mites

Fungus mutation and fungus mites are the two natural disasters which threaten a collection of dermatophyte fungi. On a small scale infestations with fungus mites rival the plagues of Egypt. Three effective steps can be taken: 1) Add dieldrin to all culture media, 2) Seal all culture tubes without fail by rimming the lip with mucilage and gluing on a piece of Ross optical lens tissue* (not lens paper), 3) Place brown paper sprayed with a chlordane containing insecticide on the mite infested shelves.

fungus mite

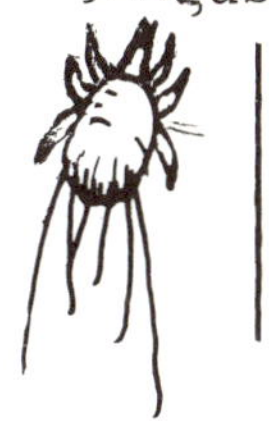

* Delaware Scientific Laboratories, Inc., P.O. Box 5107, Wilmington, Delaware 19808. (Hansen & Snyder, 1939. Science 89:350.)

To Maintain Cultures in a Dormant State

1) Lyophilize microaleuriospores in double strength skim milk (Difco). This is also a good way of selectively killing mites in a culture.

2) Preserve aleuriospores at room temperature in small, well rinsed, tight vials of glass distilled water (a simple method of keeping a source of inocula in a state unchanged by mutation).

3) Some fungi, such as T. mentagrophytes can be stored for relatively long periods (6 months) in the refrigerator. Others such as E. floccosum are killed in the refrigerator overnight. Sporulating dermatophytes may be grown on freezing agar and stored in the deep freeze. Some cultures may be kept viable under sterile mineral oil at room temperature, but become pleomorphic and lose their original characteristics.

4) Cultures of non-sporulating parasitic dermatophytes usually cannot be maintained by these methods. However, fungi in infected clinical material, such as hairs, scales, and nails, particularly if they contain arthrospores, have a better chance of remaining viable, as do fungi grown in soil-hair cultures, when dry or preserved by the above methods.

To Prepare Dead Cultures for Study

For learning to recognize cultures, cultures grown in bottles may be preserved by killing with a few drops of formaldhyde introduced into the bottle without wetting the fungus. After permitting the excess water to evaporate seal the bottles tightly. For scientific herbarium purposes, slide cultures or portions of agar cultures may be dried and preserved in vials.

Mailing Cultures in Transparent Cellophane Tape

A convenient method of airmailing dermatophyte cultures in a letter envelope has been devised by F. M. Rush-Munro (figure 8).

(1) Fix tape strip A to a piece of note paper.
(2) Place a fragment of dermatophyte culture on the surface of strip A.
(3) Fasten a cut square of tape (B) to a second tape strip (C), sticky surfaces together.
(4) Fasten strip C over strip A in the form of a cross. The specimen thus sealed in a pocket between the non-sticky surfaces of strips A and the tape square B. Infected hairs and skin scrapings can also be mailed in this way.

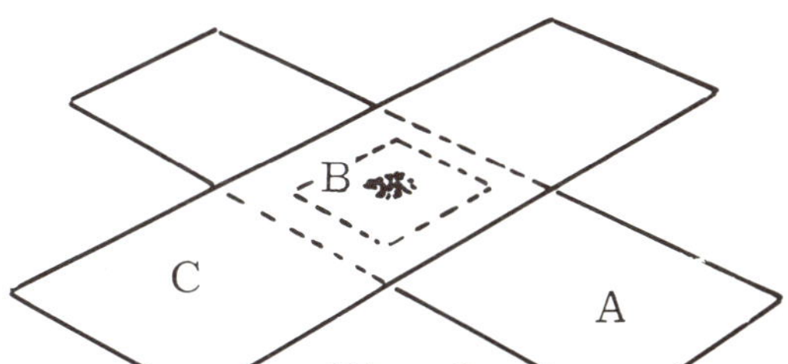

Fig. 8

TO ISOLATE DERMATOPHYTES FROM SOIL

Hair Bait Technique - Moisten the soil samples in petri dishes with sterile distilled water, and sprinkle with chopped autoclaved horse or prepubertal human hair*, which serves as a bait and becomes colonized by dermatophytes and other keratinophilic fungi present in the soil. It is advisable to add cycloheximide (500 μg/ml) and antibacterial antibiotics. A peptone dextrose agar medium designated SAB-PSA^2 by G. F. Orr (Bull. Torrey Botanical Club 95, 424-431, 1968) for direct isolation of Gymnoascaceae and related fungi from soil contains 10,000 units of penicillin, 1 mg of streptomycin, and 2 mg cycloheximide (Actidione) per ml. Similar high concentrations may be used to wet the soil in soil hair plates (Orr, G. F., Sabouraudia 7, 129-134, 1969). DTM and its antibiotic components have as yet not been explored for isolating dermatophytes from soil.

* baboon hair, hedghog quills, defatted wool (Pugh, G. J. F. Sabouraudia 5, 49-53, 1966), and chicken feathers have also been used in special circumstances.

Enrichment of Soil with Keratinous Substrates - (Somerville, D. A. and Marples, M. J., 1967, Sabouraudia 6:70-76). Addition of sterile cowhorn shavings to soil (in a plastic bag) and incubation for 14 days at environmental temperature selectively increased subsequent recovery of M. gypseum from the soil by the hair bait technique. This technique probably favors some keratinophilic fungi more than others and alters the balance of keratinophilic fungi initially present in the soil.

Isolation of Dermatophytes from Fur and Feathers - Geophilic dermatophytes and related keratinophilic fungi are commonly isolated from the fur of mammals and feathers of birds, in the absence of visible signs of skin infection or hair parasitism. Brush (or comb) the fur and inoculate the brushings on DTM; or plant hair samples directly on DTM; or first soak them in cycloheximide and antibiotic solution (see PSA^2 composition above). The number of keratinophilic fungi recovered from animal fur tends to increase with the number of individual hair sampled, regardless of whether they are from the same animal or different animals. The specific association of the red form of T. terrestre with hedgehog quills may be exceptional (see also M. persicolor). A partly different group of keratinophilic fungus species are commonly isolated from the feathers of birds (Reese, R. G., 1967, Sabouraudia 6:19-28).

To Isolate Dermatophytes from Other Fomites - A selective medium such as DTM is necessary.

References -

Ajello, L. and Getz, M.E., 1954. Recovery of Dermatophytes from Shoes and Shower Stalls, J. Invest. Derm., 22:17-21.

Gentles, J.C., 1957. Athlete's Foot Fungi on Floors of Communal Bathing Places, Brit. Med. J., i:746-748.

Mackenzie, D.W.R., 1961. The Extra-Human Occurrence of Trichophyton tonsurans var. sulfureum in a Residential School, Sabouraudia, 1:58-64.

Taplin, D., Allen, A.M., and Mertz, P.M., 1970. Experience With a New Indicator Medium (DTM) For the Isolation of Dermatophyte Fungi, Proc. Internat. Symp. Mycoses, Washington, D.C., Pan American Health Organization, Publication Number 205.

Identifying Mating Types with Arthroderma simii Mating Types - (Stockdale, P., 1968, Sabouraudia 6:176-181). Inoculate the culture to be typed on one half of two petri dishes of dextrose peptone agar and inoculate the opposing halves with the two mating types of A. simii. The mating type is revealed by the proliferation of white fluffy hyphae, often with formation of ascocarp initials (Fig. 9, page 118), which occurs when the unknown mating type makes physical contact with the thallus of A. simii of the opposite mating type. After the mating types are identified test mating can be arranged between opposite mating types to obtain ascocarps (see below). Failure to react with A. simii may be encountered with certain dermatophytes. Its significance is unknown.

Demonstrating Ascospores, The Perfect State of Dermatophytes - Inoculate (1) soil-hair plates or (2) oatmeal-salt agar plates with two different strains of dermatophyte. If the strains are opposite mating types of the same species (see above) ascocarps containing ascospores usually develop within a month. To identify an unknown culture as a described species of Nannizzia or Arthroderma, perform test matings with cultures obtained from the germination of single ascospores of the known fungus. These type (or tester) strains can be obtained from stock collections (4).

Some dermatophytes, such as N. gypsea and A. simii, produce ascospores readily. Some, such as N. persicolor, not so readily. Various factors have been described as influencing ascocarp production. Among these is the soil used (garden soil, unautoclaved, containing rusty iron, etc.), pH, and temperature. See references listed on pages 72-73 for techniques in application to different ascigerous species.

(1) Soil-Hair Plates consist of autoclaved soil, moistened with sterile water, and sprinkled with chopped, autoclaved horse hair or prepubertal human hair.

(2) Oatmeal-Salts Agar, Formula E (Weitzman, I. and Silva-Hutner, M., 1967, Sabouraudia 5:335-340), is as effective as soil-hair substrates.

Distilled water	1000 ml	$NaNO_3$	1.0 gm
$MgSO_4 \cdot 7\ H_2O$	1 gm	Beech-Nut* Baby Oatmeal	10 gm
KH_4PO_4	0.5 g	Agar Agar	10 gm

Adjust pH to 5.6 without NaOH and autoclave (127°C, 20 minutes).
*Beech-Nut, Inc., New York 10016, U.S.A.

(4) Tester strains of most ascigerous dermatophytes can be obtained from: Centraalbureau voor Schimmelcultures Baarn, Oosterstraat 1, Baarn, Netherlands and/or American Type Culture Collection, 12301 Parklawn Drive, Rockwell, Maryland 20852 U.S.A. For others, see original references cited on pages 72 and 73.

Isolation of Single Ascospores - Without a micromanipulator (de Fonbrune) this is tedious. Manual technique consists in isolating single ascospores on an agar surface or in agar blocks under the microscope and subculturing them before or after germination.

Ascigerous State - Cont.

The ascocarps of dermatophytes are spherical structures about 500 microns in diameter which become yellowish or brownish when the ascospores mature. The asci are fragile and difficult to see intact. The ascospores, eight per ascus, are small (1 to 3 microns) and generally lenticular in shape. The outer layer of the ascocarps consists of a mesh-like cortex composed of the peridial hyphae.

Fig. 9

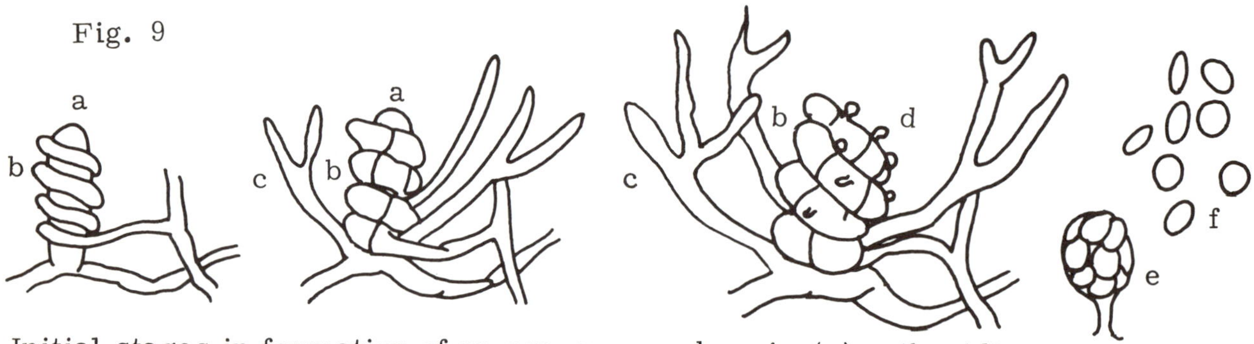

Initial stages in formation of an ascocarp and asci: (a) antheridium, (b) archigonium, (c) peridial hyphae arising from antheridium, (d) pre-ascigerous "croziers" arising from archigonium, (e) ascus, (f) ascospores.

Reference:

Weitzman, I., Allderdice, P.W., Silva-Hutner, M., and Miller, O.J., 1968. Sabouraudia, 6:232-237.

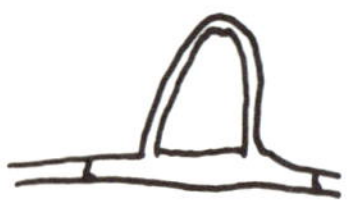

earlier stage in formation of the antheridium. Structures of this type may also be found in cultures of non-ascigerous dermatophytes, such as T. rubrum.

Illustration On Cover

Outgrowth of the saprophytic phase of Microsporum canis from a plucked, parasitized hair in a slide culture. The macro- and microaleuriospores of dermatophytes are never formed in vivo, in parasitized hair or stratum corneum, but are formed promptly in vitro. The drawing is somewhat simplified and diagrammatic.

GLOSSARY OF TERMS AND TAXONOMIC CATEGORIES

aleuriospore - a spore forming and disarticulating as described on page 2 (Barron, G. L. "The Genera of Hyphomycetes from Soil". The Williams & Wilkins Co., Baltimore, 1968).

alleles - genes which occupying the same chromosome locus are mutually exclusive in the haploid state.

anthropophilic - parasitic principally or exclusively on man.

Aphanoascus - a genus in the Cephalothecaceae including the perfect state of C. indicum, and the coprophilic fungus, A. fulvescens, (Cooke) Apinis, 1968, also sometimes isolated from soil-hair plates, and as a contaminant from skin (ref., pg. 72).

appressed - aerial hyphae lying flat.

arthroaleuriospore - a catenulate spore type, forming and disarticulating as an aleuriospore (Orr, Kuehn, and Plunkett, Canad. J. Botany 41, 1457-1480). In the fungi described in this manual three types occur: 1) mycelial (alternate arthrospores),  2) catenulate aleuriospores,  3) modified macroaleuriospores.

Arthroderma - a genus in the Gymnoascaceae defined by the cells of the peridial hyphae which are dumb-bell shaped, with or without lateral protuberances. All known species have either Trichophyton or Chrysosporium aleuriospore states.

arthrospore - spore or segment produced by fragmentation of septate hyphae. Produced by dermatophytes in culture and in hair (arthroaleuriospores?), nails, and epidermal scales. 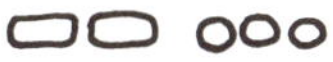

ascigerous - productive of ascospores (and associated structures of the perfect state of the Ascomycetes).

ascocarp - a structure composed of more or less modified hyphae partially or completely enclosing the ascigerous hyphae and asci.

Ascomycetes - fungi in which the perfect state is manifest by production of asci and ascospores.

ascospore - genetically segregated haploid spores of the perfect state in the Ascomycetes (see pgs. 8, 116).

ascus (plural asci) - sack-like cell containing mature ascospores.

asymmetric - in reference to 1) peridial hyphae in which the cells have a greater protuberance on one side than the other, and 2) macroaleuriospores which are somewhat curved.

attachment scar - the base of an aleuriospore, marking its point of detachment from the parent hypha.

balloon forms- microaleuriospores tending to become enlarged and spherical.

beak - a terminal knob or nipple-shaped tip of a macroaleuriospore.

bullet-shaped - 

carpet-like - short, dense pile of aerial hyphae.

catenulate - formed in chains.

Cephalothecaceae - Ascomycetes in which the ascocarp is intermediate between Gymnoascaceae and Eurotiaceae.

chlamydospores - swollen, thick-walled hyphal elements. 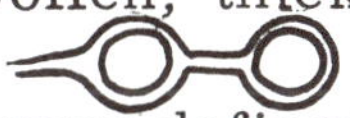

Chrysosporium - a genus defined by having either smooth or echinulate, single-celled aleuriospores ranging in size from microaleuriospores to considerably larger. Ascigerous species are in the genera Arthroderma, Ctenomyces, Aphanoascus, and other genera not considered in this manual.

cigar-shaped - 

clavate - club-shaped.

cleistothecium - a spherical ascocarp without a defined opening (commonly used to include the more basket-like ascocarps of Nannizzia and Arthroderma).

club-shaped - 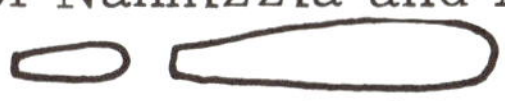

coils - filamentous terminal hyphae, coiled like springs.

colony - a group of organisms originating from a single inoculum, applicable to bacterial and yeast colonies, but because of the continuous nature of the filamentous fungus organism not as descriptive of fungi.

conidia - lateral or terminal spores which are shed from the hyphae (may be used generally to include, or restricted to exclude, aleuriospores).

conidial state - the vegetative, spore forming mycelia of a perfect fungus or its mating types.

conidiophore - hyphal structures more or less differentiated for the production of spores.

cottony - loose, coarse, or tufted aerial hyphae.

Ctenomyces - a genus in the Gymnoascaceae defined by comb-like peridial appendages.

cycloheximide - (Actidione) an antibiotic preventing protein synthesis in eukaryotic cells (including fungi).

dermatophytes - as used in this manual: fungi of the genera Microsporum, Trichophyton, and Epidermophyton, regardless of pathogenicity.

dichotomous - branched by repeated forks.

distorted - angularly misshapen.

downy - covered with short, sparse to dense aerial hyphae.

dumbbell-shaped - 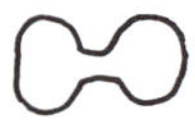

dysgonic - slow growing variant (in M. canis and M. audouinii).

echinulate - spiny surfaced (for scanning electronmicrographs of macroaleuriospores, see Ho et al 1970. Sabouraudia, 7:270-272).

ectothrix - parasitism of hair with vegetative hyphae inside the hair and arthrospores principally on the surface of the hair.

endothrix - parasitism of hair with formation of arthrospores inside the hair.

Epidermophyton - a genus defined by having multiseptate club-shaped macroaleuriospores but no microaleuriospores. The single species is E. floccosum.

eukaryotic - having a membrane-bound nucleus and other characteristics of protozoan, plant, animal, and fungus cells, as opposed to bacterial (prokaryotic) cells).

Eurotiaceae - Ascomycetes in which the ascocarp consists of a compact pseudoparenchymal cortex, as opposed to a loose basket-like interlacing of filamentous hyphae.

filiform - slender and filament-like. 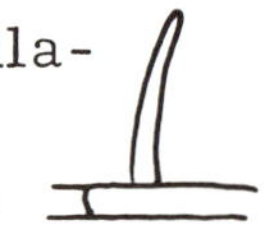

fluffy - a dense, deep pile of aerial hyphae.

Fungi Imperfecti - a taxonomic designation for fungi with no known perfect state.

fuzzy - near glabrous, but with a short pile of aerial hyphae.

geophilic - occurring principally as a saprobe in soil.

glabrous - without or almost without aerial hyphae.

granular - macroscopically coarsely powdery or roughened (in this manual not synonymous with heavily powdery).

griseofulvin - an antibiotic with a unique degree of activity against dermatophytes and related fungi; action probably on microtubules involved in mitosis and morphogenesis of eukaryotic cells.

Gymnoascaceae - Ascomycetes in which the ascocarp is loose and basket-like, composed of somewhat specialized (frequently ornamented) peridial hyphae. (Apinis, A. E. "Revision of British Gymnoascaceae." Commonwealth Mycological Institute; Kew, Surrey, England, 1964).

heaped - elevated and mound-like (usually more or less glabrous).

heavily powdery - a thick layer of spores on surface of the thallus.

heterothallic - requiring copulation between the mycelia of two strains for the production of ascospores.

hour-glass shaped - constricted in midlength.

hyphae - a filamentous element or strand of fungus mycelium.

imperfect fungus - see Fungi Imperfecti.

intercalary - inserted in a mycelial filament, as opposed to terminal.

knob - see beak.

lanceolate - narrow and tapered to a point.

lateral - produced along the sides of the hypha, as opposed to terminal.

lenticular - double convex, as the seed of a lentil.

macroaleuriospore - an aleuriospore-type with predominantly two or more chambers (cells)

Malbranchea - a genus of soil fungi defined by having as the principal spore type arthroaleuriospores (or alternate arthrospores) in simple branches similar to those seen in some species and isolates of Trichophyton and Chrysosporium and suggestive of the fungus Coccidioides immitis. See also Auxarthron (Orr, Kuehn, and Plunkett, 1963, Canad. J. Botany 41, 1439-1456), and Oidiodendron.

megaspore - Sabouraud's term for large spored ectothrix (T. verrucosum).

microaleuriospore - a type of aleuriospore consisting predominantly of one cell, and of small size (usually less than 5μ maximum axis).

microides - Sabouraud's term for small ectothrix in chains (T. mentagrophytes).

Microsporum - a genus defined by having echinulate macroaleuriospores (predominantly spindle-shaped), and smooth microaleuriospores.

Mycelia Sterilia - taxonomic designation for filamentous fungi which fail to produce spores of any kind.

mycelium - filamentous mat or vegetative whole of a fungus.

nail-head hyphae - hyphae with expanded, branched tips as in T. schoenleinii.

Nannizzia - a genus in the Gymnoascaceae defined by cells of the peridial hyphae, which are phalangiform, but otherwise similar to Arthroderma. All known species have Microsporum aleuriospore states.

nodular organ - a knot of hyphae somewhat resembling preascigerous copulation of hyphae. 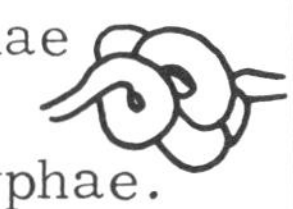

oat-shaped - ovoid and somewhat pointed at both ends. 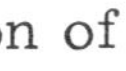

obovoid-egg shaped - attached at small end. 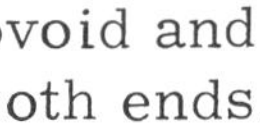

Oidiodendron - a genus characterized by usually somewhat pigmented arthroaleuriospores produced on erect, tree-like conidiophores (Barron, G. L., 1962, Canad. J. Botany 40, pt. 1, 589-607). Perfect forms are in Gymnoascaceae.

pectinate hypha - a comb-like hyphal element. 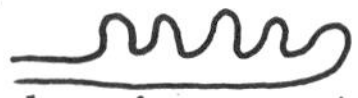

pedicellate - having a stalk or short supporting hyphae. 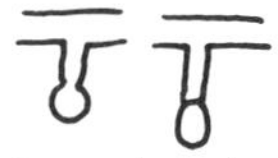

peg-shaped - 

perfect state - a state in which nuclear fusion associated with a sexual process occurs (followed in the Ascomycetes by production of ascospores).

perforating organ - see pages 5 and 109.

peridial hyphae - thick, claw-like hyphae which entangle to form the ascocarp.

phalangiform - shaped like finger bones. 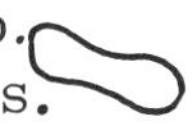

propagule - structure found in T. proliferans (see page 67).

pycnidia - an ascocarp-like structure containing vegetative spores rather than ascospores.

pyriform - pear-shaped. 

raceme - a wand or plume-like branching fructification.

reflexive - branching backward.

spindle-shaped - 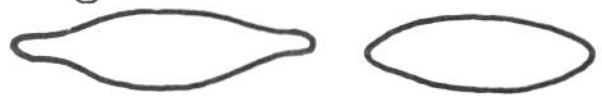

spiral hyphae - see coils.

tadpole-shaped - 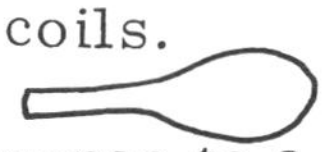

terminal - with reference to a single spore or branching cluster of aleuriospores produced at the end (or end portion) of a hypha.

thallus - the fungus organism considered as a branching continuum starting from a germinal spore or some initial center of growth.

Trichophyton - a genus defined by having smooth macroaleuriospores (predominantly cylindrical) and smooth microaleuriospores.

twiggy - branching with an angular, somewhat stiff appearance.

uncinate - branching backward in a hooked fashion from a principal hypha.

verticillate - branched in whorls of three or more.

zoophilic - parasitic principally on animals other than man.

INDEX OF SYNONYMS

The names chosen for this short synonomy have persisted in the recent literature and in certain books, or have only recently been revised.

Achorion (obsolete) - see Microsporum and Trichophyton
gallinae (21 T. (M?) gallinae)
gypseum (23 M. gypseum)
quinckeanum (40 T. mentagrophytes)
schoenleinii (59 T. schoenleinii)

Anixiopsis stercoraria (118 A. fulvescens)

Arthroderma benhamii (40 A. benhamiae)
lenticulare (33 A. lenticularum)

Ctenomyces (only C. serratus in this genus) - see Trichophyton and Microsporum
asteroides (40 T. mentagrophytes)
denticulatus (40 T. mentagrophytes)
granulosus (um) (40 T. mentagrophytes)
interdigitale (40 T. mentagrophytes)
persicolor (27 M. persicolor)
radiolans (40 T. mentagrophytes)
radians (40 T. mentagrophytes)
terrestre (33 T. terrestre)
trichophyticus (33 T. terrestre)

Endodermophyton - see Trichophyton

Endotrichophyton - see Trichophyton

Epidermophyton (only E. floccosum in this genus)
cruris (62 E. floccosum)
indicum (61 T. concentricum)
inguinale (62 E. floccosum)
interdigitale (40 T. mentagrophytes)
radiosulcatum (25 M. fulvum)
rubrum (50 T. rubrum)
tropicale (61 T. concentricum)

Favotrichophyton - see Trichophyton

Gymnoascus (no dermatophyte in this genus)
gypseum (23 N. gypsea)

Keratinophyton terreum (eus) (71 A. terreus)

Keratomyces ajelloi (31 T. ajelloi)
longifusus (31 T. longifusus)

Langeronia - see Trichophyton

Microsporon - see Microsporum

Microsporum album (19 M. ferrugineum)
aureum (19 M. ferrugineum)
caninum (13 M. canis)
duboisii (23 M. gypseum)
equinum (13 M. canis)
felineum (eus) (13 M. canis)
gallinae (21 T. (M?) gallinae)
japonicum (19 M. ferrugineum)
langeronii (16 M. audouinii)
lanosum (13 M. canis)
obesum (13 M. canis)
orientale (19 M. ferrugineum)
quinckeanum (40 T. mentagrophytes)
rivalierii (16 M. audouinii)
simie (13 M. canis)

Nannizzia cajetana (29 N. cajetani)

Pinoyella simii (38 T. simii)

Sabouraudites - see Microsporum

Thallomicrosporon kuehnii (25 M. fulvum)

Trichophyton accuminatum (52 T. tonsurans)
album (19 M. ferrugineum or 47 T. verrucosum)
asteroides (40 T. mentagrophytes)
cerebriforme (52 T. tonsurans)
crateriforme (52 T. tonsurans)
discoides (47 T. verrucosum)
epilans (52 T. tonsurans)
evolceanui (71 C. evolceanui)
faviforme (47 T. verrucosum)
ferrugineum (19 M. ferrugineum)
fumatum (52 T. tonsurans)
gallopavium (21 T. (M?) gallinae?)
glabrum (54 T. violaceum)
granulosum (us) (40 T. mentagrophytes
gypseum (40 T. mentagrophytes)
indicum (71 C. indicum)
interdigitale (40 T. mentagrophytes)
kagewaense (54 T. violaceum)
Kaufman-Wolf (40 T. mentagrophytes)
kuryangei (49 T. megninii)

LIST OF EXCLUDED SPECIES

Some of the following species appear to be based on mixed cultures (see Ajello, L., 1968, Sabouraudia 6:147-159). In others the original description is not adequate (and the original cultures no longer available for study) so that the species cannot be evaluated.

Epidermophyton album Szathmary, 1940: Arch. Derm. Syph. Wien 181, 192-203.
Favomicrosporon pinetti Benedek, 1967: Mycopath. Mycol. Appl. 31, 81-143.
Microsporum cornua-bovis, 1954: Galli & Conferi Ann. Fac. Med. Vet. Tovino, 4, 169-181.
Trichophyton citreum Szathmary, 1935: Orv. Hétil. 79, 1264-1266.
T. fluviale Szathmary, 1940: Arch. Derm. Syph. Wien 181:192-203.
T. gallopavium Metiano, Lucas & Drouhet, 1966: Mycopath. Mycol. Appl., 30, 22-30. Possibly T. (M?) gallinae - see Gordon and Little, 1968 (reference page 22).
T. lipoterum Kominami, 1961: Jap. J. Med. Mycol, 2, 38-41.
T. otae Dowding, 1944: Canad. J. Res., 22, 67-77.
T. pervesi Catanei, 1937: Arch. Inst. Pasteur, 15, 265-270.
T. radiocosum Catanei, 1937: Ibid.
Veronaia audouinii Benedek, 1961: Mycopath. Mycol. Appl., 14, 101-122.
V. castellani Benedek, 1961: Ibid.
V. felineii Benedek, 1961: Ibid.

INDEX OF SPECIES